Ectopic Pregnancy and Prenatal Diagnosis

Edited by Wei Wu, Qiuqin Tang, Panagiotis Tsikouras, Werner Rath, Georg-Friedrich Von Tempelhoff and Nikolaos Nikolettos

Published in London, United Kingdom

Ectopic Pregnancy and Prenatal Diagnosis
http://dx.doi.org/10.5772/intechopen.98077
Edited by Wei Wu, Qiuqin Tang, Panagiotis Tsikouras, Werner Rath, Georg-Friedrich Von Tempelhoff and Nikolaos Nikolettos

Contributors
Radu Vladareanu, Hadi Rahimian, Ramona Ana Maria Rahimian, Subrat Panda, Ananya Das, Anusuya Sharma, Prateeti Baruah, Kaushiki Singh, Maged Shendy, Sonia Abhishek, Lisa Dhege, Ibrahim Alatwi, Sergio Rosales-Ortiz, Tammy Barrón Martinez, Jose Fugarolas Marin, Alejandra Vega León, Rogelio Apolo Aguado Pérez, Carlos Augusto De La Cruz Vázquez, Janeth Marquez-Acosta, Smarth Santacruz Baez, Afaf Filimban, Haya Aljurayfani, Hessa Alkharif, Fatmah Alamri, Hadeel Alkhelb, Mohammed Albugnah, Jawaher Alsahabi, Ghadeer L. Aljahdali, Bahati Johnson, Marina Sica, Carlotta Plessi, Francesco Molinaro, Artúr Beke, Aténé Simonyi, Virág Bartek, Wei Wu, Tong Wang, Jiahe Xu, Lin Wang, Qiuqin Tang, Xiumin Cui, Yan Yan, Brinda Sabu, Vidyalekshmy Ranganayaki, Ryan Holman

First published in London, United Kingdom, 2022 by IntechOpen
IntechOpen is the global imprint of INTECHOPEN LIMITED, registered in England and Wales, registration number: 11086078, 5 Princes Gate Court, London, SW7 2QJ, United Kingdom

British Library Cataloguing-in-Publication Data
A catalogue record for this book is available from the British Library

Additional hard and PDF copies can be obtained from orders@intechopen.com

Ectopic Pregnancy and Prenatal Diagnosis
Edited by Wei Wu, Qiuqin Tang, Panagiotis Tsikouras, Werner Rath, Georg-Friedrich Von Tempelhoff and Nikolaos Nikolettos
p. cm.
Print ISBN 978-1-80355-840-0
Online ISBN 978-1-80355-841-7
eBook (PDF) ISBN 978-1-80355-842-4

Meet the editors

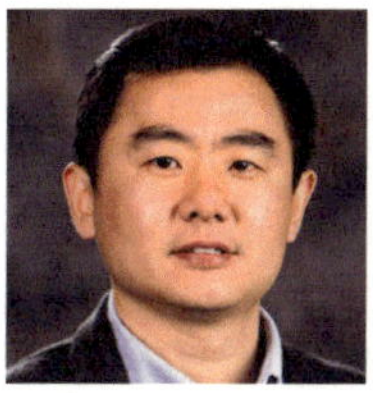

Wei Wu is assistant to the Dean at the School of Public Health, and Professor and Associate Department Chair of the Department of Toxicology at Nanjing Medical University, China, where he received his Ph.D. in toxicology in 2012. He was a guest researcher at the National Institute of Environmental Health Sciences (NIEHS) between 2017 and 2018. He is the PI of the State Key Laboratory of Reproductive Medicine and the PI of the Key Laboratory of Modern Toxicology at the Ministry of Education. Dr. Wu is a member of several national and international societies in the fields of human reproduction and toxicology and has received awards from many national societies for the originality and quality of his projects. Dr. Wu has authored 78 peer-reviewed papers in international journals. He has edited four books and collaborated on 10 books, 11 patents and in the organization of three international conferences. He is a reviewer for 104 international journals.

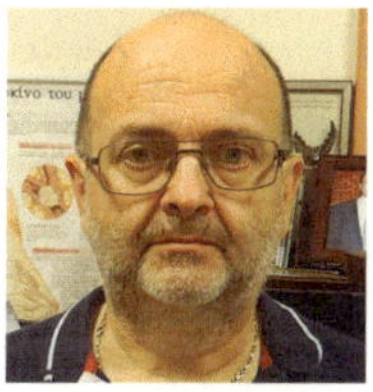

Panagiotis Tsikouras is a specialist in obstetrics and gynecology, perinatal medicine, and contraception at the School of Medicine, Democritus University of Thrace, Greece. He is also head of the Family Planning Centre and Gynecological Cytology Laboratory at the same university. Dr. Tsikouras is a fellow of the International Academy of Clinical and Applied Thrombosis/Hemostasis. His scientific activities focus on pediatric and adolescent medicine, gynecological oncology, and high-risk pregnancies. He is a reviewer for several international journals and has numerous scientific publications to his credit, including papers and book chapters. He has also contributed to international and national guidelines on coagulation and thrombosis in obstetrics and gynecology.

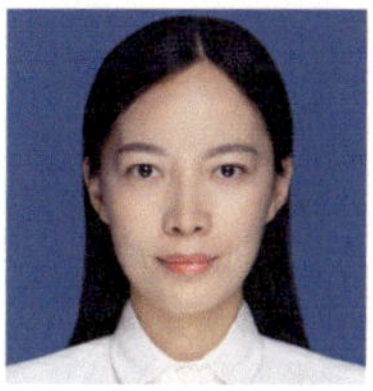

Qiuqin Tang is an associate chief physician of the Women's Hospital of Nanjing Medical University (Nanjing Maternity and Child Health Care Hospital). Her research interests include genetic and epigenetic risk factors in reproductive and developmental health. She has authored 29 papers in international journals such as *EBioMedicine*, *Environmental Pollution*, *Clinical Epigenetics*, *Molecular Human Reproduction*, and *European Journal of Endocrinology*. She has collaborated on four books and three patents. She is the editor-in-chief of the *Journal of Woman's Reproductive Health*.

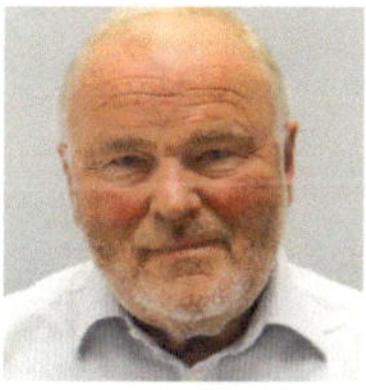

Werner Rath is a specialist in obstetrics and gynecology, gynecological oncology, perinatal medicine and hemostaseology. Currently a professor of gynecology and obstetrics at Kiel University, he previously led the Department of Gynecology and Obstetrics at University Hospital, Aachen. He holds an honorary doctorate from the University of Alexandroupolis. He has received the Staude-Pfannenstiel Award of the North German Society of Gynaecology & Obstetrics, the Maternity Award of the German Society of Perinatal Medicine, Berlin, and the Harald-Bräutigam Award, Hamburg. His citable research publications date from 1977. He is a reviewer for numerous journals and, in addition to his publications and 13 book chapters, was chief editor of the German *Journal of Obstetrics & Gynaecology* (*Geburtshilfe und Frauenheilkunde*).

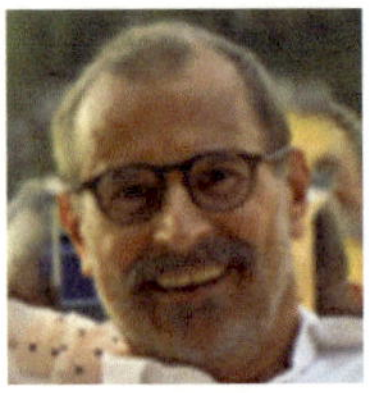

Georg-Friedrich von Tempelhoff, FCATH, is a specialist in obstetrics and gynecology, gynecological oncology, perinatal medicine and hemostaseology. He is head of the Department of Gynecology and Obstetrics at St. Vinzenz Hospital, Hanau and head of the Institute for Thrombosis and Coagulation Disorders in Gynecology and Obstetrics, Hausen. He was educated at the Justus-Liebig University in Giessen, receiving his doctorate in medicine in 1993. He became a consultant in obstetrics and gynecology in 1996. He completed his habilitation at the Johannes-Gutenberg University Mainz in 2007 and was appointed extracurricular professor at the Julius-Maximilians-Universität Würzburg in 2015. He is a fellow of the International Academy of Clinical and Applied Thrombosis / Hemostasis. His research focus is on hemostaseological and hemorheological disorders in women with miscarriages, pre-eclampsia and thrombosis. He is a reviewer for numerous journals and, in addition to his publications and book chapters, has contributed to international and national guidelines on coagulation and thrombosis in gynecology.

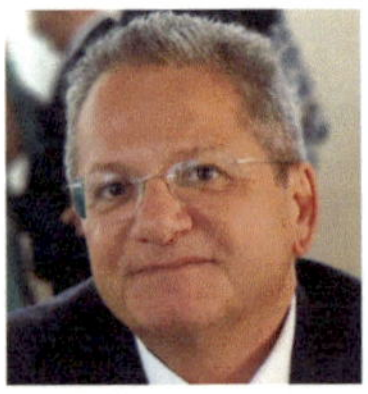

Nikolettos Nikos has been a professor of obstetrics, gynecology and assisted reproduction at Democritus University of Thrace, since 2018, and has managed the Obstetrics and Gynecology Clinic since 2019. From 2007 to 2011 he was a director of the In-Vitro Fertilization Unit of the University Regional General Hospital, Alexandroupolis. From 2012 to 2018 he was director of the Laboratory of Reproductive Physiology and Artificial Fertilization. He has more than 100 publications in international journals and has delivered many lectures by invitation to international and Greek conferences.

Contents

Preface

Ectopic pregnancy is an important cause of morbidity and mortality worldwide, occurring in approximately 2% of all pregnancies, and leading to 2.7%–5% of maternal deaths in developed countries, mainly from ectopic pregnancy rupture. It is associated with abdominal pain and transvaginal bleeding, and its prevalence in emergency services is 18%. However, with early diagnosis, complications can be avoided. Prenatal screening categorizing pregnancies as high or low risk to prevent maternal complications, and screening the fetus for aneuploidies, anomalies, and growth abnormalities, provides clinicians with evidence for intrauterine treatment or selective termination of pregnancy, and enables the time and mode of safe delivery to be determined and an optimal perinatal outcome to be achieved.

The book is divided into three sections: Diagnosis and Medical Management of Ectopic Pregnancy (Chapters 1–5), Fetal Malformation (Chapters 6–8), and Prenatal Diagnosis and Screening (Chapters 9–11).

Chapter 1 presents a case of heterotopic pregnancy and discusses the endoscopic management of ectopic pregnancy, including incidence and risk factors, clinical presentation and diagnosis, differential diagnosis, treatments, and outcomes.

Chapter 2, on gynecological endoscopy, discusses the endoscopic management of ectopic pregnancy, tubal pregnancy, interstitial or horn pregnancy, ovarian pregnancy, abdominal pregnancy, heterotopic pregnancy, cervical pregnancy, niche, cesarean scar pregnancy, and fertility and ectopic pregnancy.

Chapter 3 reviews the medical management of ectopic pregnancy. Topics addressed include the pharmacology of methotrexate, selection criteria, administration, success, and contraindications for methotrexate. Post-treatment pain, post-methotrexate Anti-D, the role in pregnancy of unknown location, the role of methotrexate in ectopic post-surgical management, and the role of methotrexate in challenging non-tubal ectopic pregnancies are all discussed.

Chapter 4 discusses the diagnosis of ectopic pregnancy, the high index of suspicion of the condition, and the importance of comprehensive training for clinicians.

Chapter 5 examines ectopic pregnancy after ipsilateral salpingectomy, focusing on the pathophysiological, diagnostic, treatment, and prevention aspects. Recurrent ectopic pregnancy in the portion of the tube remaining after ipsilateral salpingectomy has only rarely been reported.

Chapter 6 discusses the prenatal diagnosis of diaphragmatic hernia, including its classification, pathogenesis, antenatal management, postnatal management, and long-term outcomes.

Chapter 7 discusses the etiology and diagnostics of each fetal craniospinal disorder, including ultrasound diagnostics and genetic testing options.

Chapter 8 introduces aspects of spina bifida and myelomeningocele, such as etiology, pathophysiology and methods of diagnosis. The chapter also presents the indications and surgical protocols for both procedures. The author includes statistics on the cases diagnosed and operated on in the Regina Maria Maternity Hospital, Bucharest, the only center in Romania where these procedures are available.

Chapter 9 discusses advances in the application of biomarkers for prenatal diagnosis, along with associated strengths and limitations. Several representative fetal diseases are also analyzed.

Chapter 10 discusses the different screening methods which can be applied to three stages of prenatal care: the pre-pregnancy period; the inverted pyramid of care from 11 weeks till delivery; and the postnatal period.

Chapter 11 highlights common indications for the use of MRI in maternal-fetal medicine, including diagnosis and treatment. An in-depth analysis of the SARS-CoV-2 virus and pregnancy-related complications is also included.

The completion of this book would not have been possible without the efforts of numerous contributors. We would like to acknowledge the work of our co-authors. We are also grateful to Mrs. Maja Bozicevic, Mrs. Ivana Barac, and Mrs. Ana Simcic at IntechOpen for their continuing support from the inception to the completion of the book.

Wei Wu
Department of Toxicology,
School of Public Health,
Nanjing Medical University,
Nanjing, China

Panagiotis Tsikouras
Democritus University of Thrace,
Greece

Qiuqin Tang
Department of Obstetrics,
Women's Hospital of Nanjing Medical University,
Nanjing, China

Werner Rath
Kiel University,
Kiel, Germany

Georg-Friedrich Von Tempelhoff
St. Vinzenz Krankenhaus,
Hanau, Germany

Nikolaos Nikolettos
Democritus University of Thrace,
Greece

Section 1

Diagnosis and Medical Management of Ectopic Pregnancy

Chapter 1

Heterotopic Pregnancy

Bahati Johnson

Abstract

Spontaneous heterotopic pregnancy is a rare clinical and potentially dangerous condition in which intrauterine (IU) and extra-uterine pregnancies occur at the same time. It can be a life-threatening condition and can be easily missed, with the diagnosis being overlooked. A high index of suspicion is needed in women with risk factors for an ectopic pregnancy and in low-risk women with an IU gestation who have free fluid with or without an adnexal mass or in those presenting acute abdominal pain and shock. The ectopic component is usually treated surgically and the IU one is expected to continue normally. Salpingectomy is the standard surgical approach of a coexistent tubal pregnancy and should be the first line of treatment in patients with hemodynamic instability or other signs of tubal rupture. In expert hands, an unruptured ectopic pregnancy can be treated with local feticidal injection under sonographic guidance.

Keywords: heterotopic pregnancy, extrauterine pregnancy, intrauterine pregnancy

1. Introduction

Spontaneous heterotopic pregnancy is a rare clinical but a potentially dangerous phenomenon where intrauterine (IU) and extra-uterine pregnancies occur at the same time. This is a life-threatening condition and can be easily missed, with the diagnosis usually being overlooked. A high index of suspicion is needed in women with risk factors for an ectopic pregnancy and in low-risk women with an intra-uterine gestation who have free fluid with or without an adnexal mass or in those presenting acute abdominal pain and shock. The ectopic component is usually treated surgically and the IU one is expected to continue normally if it is live.

Case: *A 20-year-old woman, prime-gravid, was admitted to the gynaecology ward at 10 weeks of amenorrhea, with vaginal bleeding for 2 days, dyspnea and hypotension. Her pregnancy occurred spontaneously. Her past history did not suggest previous history of pelvic inflammatory disease, abortions, infertility or abdominal surgery or trauma. The physical examination revealed a conscious woman however with severe pallor of the palms, conjunctivae, mucous membranes of the buccal cavity and palms. She had hypotension of 75 mmHg systolic blood pressure, respiratory rate of 24 breaths per minute, SPO2 of 92%, cold sweat, and a thin thready rapid pulse of 136 beats per minute. Per abdomen did not suggest intra-abdominal haemorrhage as there was only moderate tenderness and no features of peritonism. Vaginal examination revealed active per vaginal bleeding with visible clots of fresh blood, products of conception hanging in the cervical canal. A clinical diagnosis of an incomplete abortion was made and patient was prepared for an emergency*

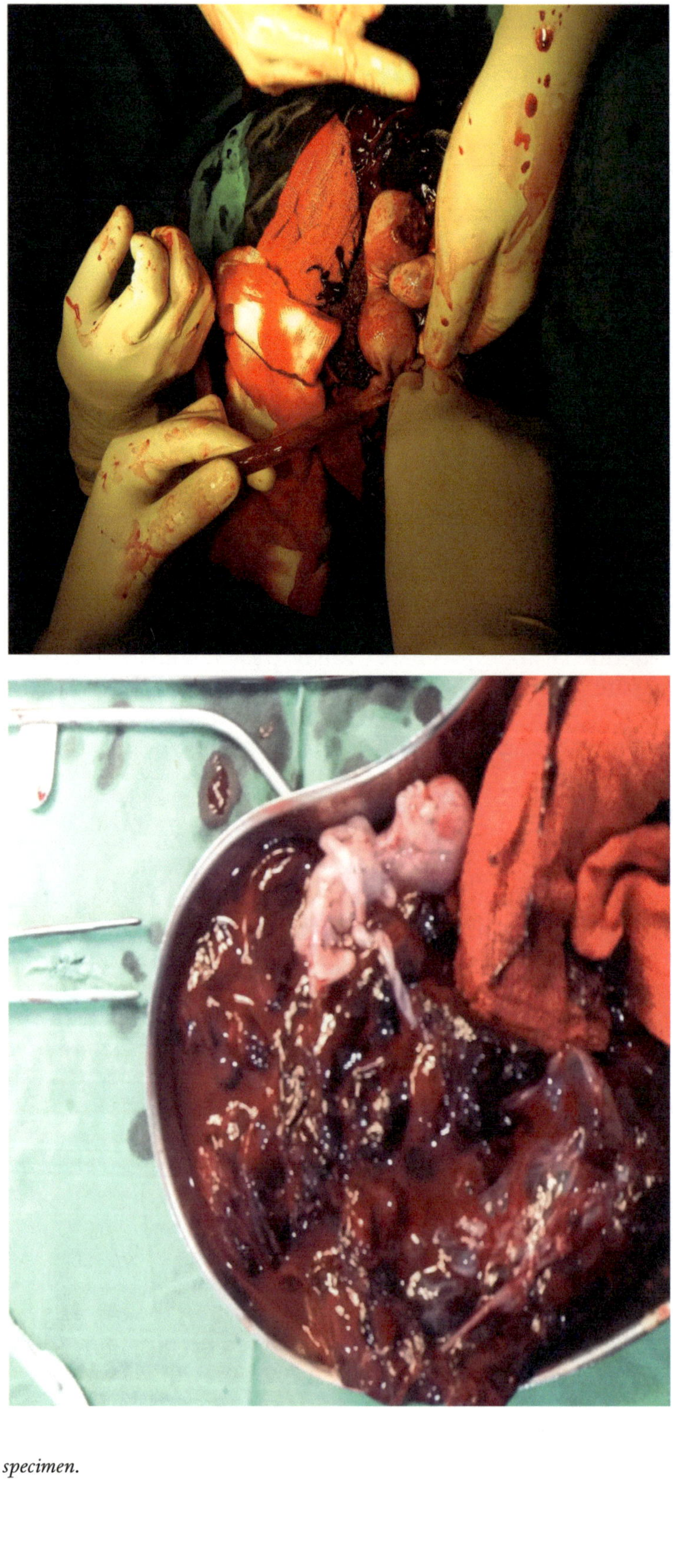

Figure 1.
Salpingectomy specimen.

uterine evacuation, which was done with a blunt curettage and curetted plenty of products of conception. Laboratory evaluation showed a normal range white blood cell count, a haematocrit of 18% and haemoglobin concentration of 6.1 g/dL, with a normal blood platelet level (390,000/mm^3), a blood urea of 44 mg/dL and a creatinine level of 1.09 mg/dL. The patient was admitted to the high dependency unit (HDU) after uterine evacuation with a continuous assessment of her airway, breathing and circulation and administration of 2.0 L of crystalloid fluids over the next 4 h. She was also given 3 units of whole blood. However her haemodynamic observations remained unstable and she developed features of acute abdomen including moderate abdominal distension with positive fluid thrill, severe tenderness with guarding and rigidity. An emergency bedside abdominal ultrasound scan (USS) was done, which demonstrated free intra-peritoneal fluid and an ill-defined right adnexal mass measuring 69.79 mm in diameter. The uterine cavity was however empty following uterine evacuation. These USS findings (free intra-peritoneal fluid and adnexal mass) in a hypovolemic-shocked patient with peritonism but no history of trauma made us think about the presence of a possible concurrent ectopic pregnancy that was not initially thought about. Also, the patient's shock did not respond to fluid resuscitation with increasing abdominal distension. Repeat complete blood count revealed further fall in the patient's haematocrit and haemoglobin concentration. The patient was thus prepared and taken to the operation theatre for an emergency exploratory laparotomy to establish and control the source of intra-abdominal haemorrhage. At laparotomy under general anaesthesia, through a sub-umbilical midline incision, revealed a ruptured right tubal gestation with active bleeding. At least 1.5 L of clots of fresh blood was evacuated from the peritoneal cavity right and left ovaries and the left tube were grossly normal. Total right tubal excision (salpingectomy) as shown in **Figure 1***, with suction of the haemoperitoneum and peritoneal lavage with saline water. Eight litres of whole blood was transfused to the patient during and after the operation. The patient recovered fully with no recorded complications. Both the tubal pregnancy and intrauterine pregnancy were confirmed at histological analysis of the salpingectomy specimen and endometrial curetting specimens that were sampled. The patient recovered uneventfully and was discharged from the hospital within 4 days.*

2. Definition

Heterotopic pregnancy is defined as the presence of multiple gestations, with one being present in the uterine cavity and the other extra-uterine, commonly in the fallopian tube and uncommonly in the cervix or ovary [1–3].

3. Incidence and risk factors

Initially described in 1708 as a postmortem discovery [4]. Under normal circumstances, with natural conception cycles, heterotopic pregnancy is an unusual occurrence with an incidence of <1/30,000 pregnancies [2, 4–6]. It accounts for 0.08% of all pregnancies [7]. The frequency of heterotopic pregnancy has increased to between 1/100 and 1/500 with assisted reproduction techniques [5, 8]. Its occurrence is 5% of conception achieved after in vitro fertilisation (IVF) [4]. Triplet heterotopic pregnancy has also been seen following natural conceptions [9]. A case, of ectopic gestation in both tubes bilaterally with an intra-uterine pregnancy has also been reported [10]. The diagnoses of heterotopic gestations are frequently made at gestation age of 5–34 weeks with 70% at 5–8 weeks, 20% at 9–10 weeks and only 10% >11 weeks of gestation [8, 11, 12].

4. Clinical presentation and diagnosis

The early detection of heterotopic pregnancy is usually very problematic due to non-specific clinical symptoms as signs of the intra-uterine pregnancy always predominate [11]. Mainly, the four cardinal clinical features common in most literature are: abdominal pain, adnexal mass, features of peritonism and an enlarged uterus [1, 11]. About 83% of heterotopic pregnancies report abdominal pain alone while 13% present with hypovolemic shock together with abdominal tenderness. More than half of the pregnant patients with heterotopic gestations do not present with

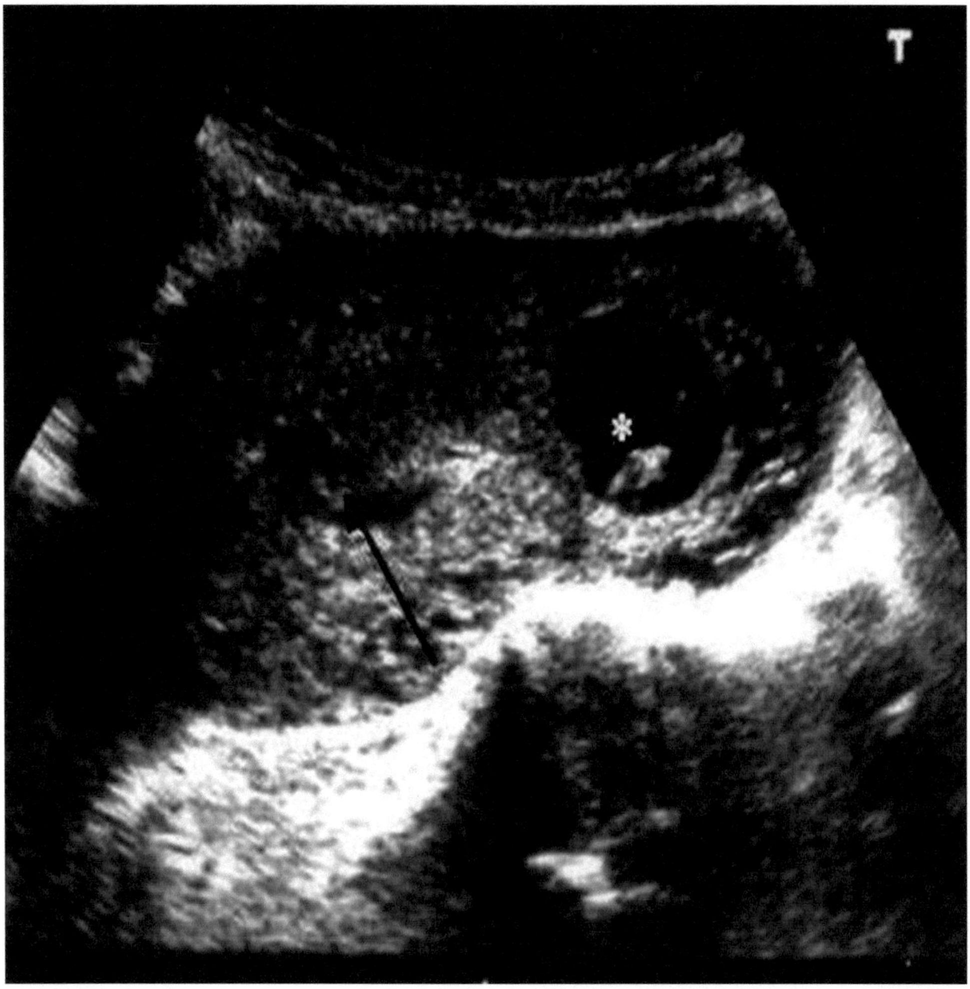

Figure 2.
Image of a trans-vaginal sonography of the uterus (transverse section) showing an intrauterine gestation (black arrow) coexisting with an ectopic cornual pregnancy (*) with a sac of 25 mm in diameter, containing an embryo with a crown rump length of 13 mm.

vaginal bleeding though it may be retrograde from the extra-uterine pregnancy due to intact endometrium of the intrauterine pregnancy [8, 13]. Increasing knowledge and skills in trans-vaginal ultrasound scanning has eased early and timely detection of heterotopic gestations. Trans-vaginal ultrasound scanning is an important tool in timely and accurate detection of heterotopic gestations. However its sensitivity in detecting heterotopic gestation is as low as 56% at 5–6 weeks [14]. Diagnosis a heterotopic gestation is confirmed at trans-vaginal sonography if there is an intra-uterine pregnancy together with an ectopic gestation (**Figure 2**) [14]. In a retrospective review of ultra-sonographic findings it was discovered that a fallopian tubal ring (an adnexal mass with a concentric echogenic rim of tissue, a gestational sac, surrounding a hypo-echoic empty center) was present in 68% of the ectopic pregnancies in which the tube had not ruptured [15]. If the pregnancy is >6 weeks, confirmation of the diagnosis is made on the presence of a cardiac activity. Sometimes, even with trans-vaginal ultrasonography, the adnexal mass is mistaken for a hemorrhagic corpus luteum or ovarian cyst, especially in ovarian hyper-stimulation [16]. In these cases, a heterotopic gestation becomes unnoticed in the presence of intra-uterine gestation. Therefore, when the levels of human chorionic gonadotropin (β-hCG) are higher for the period of gestation with an intra-uterine pregnancy, one has to find out for a possible coexistence of a tubal gestation. Occasionally, there are no concrete adnexal

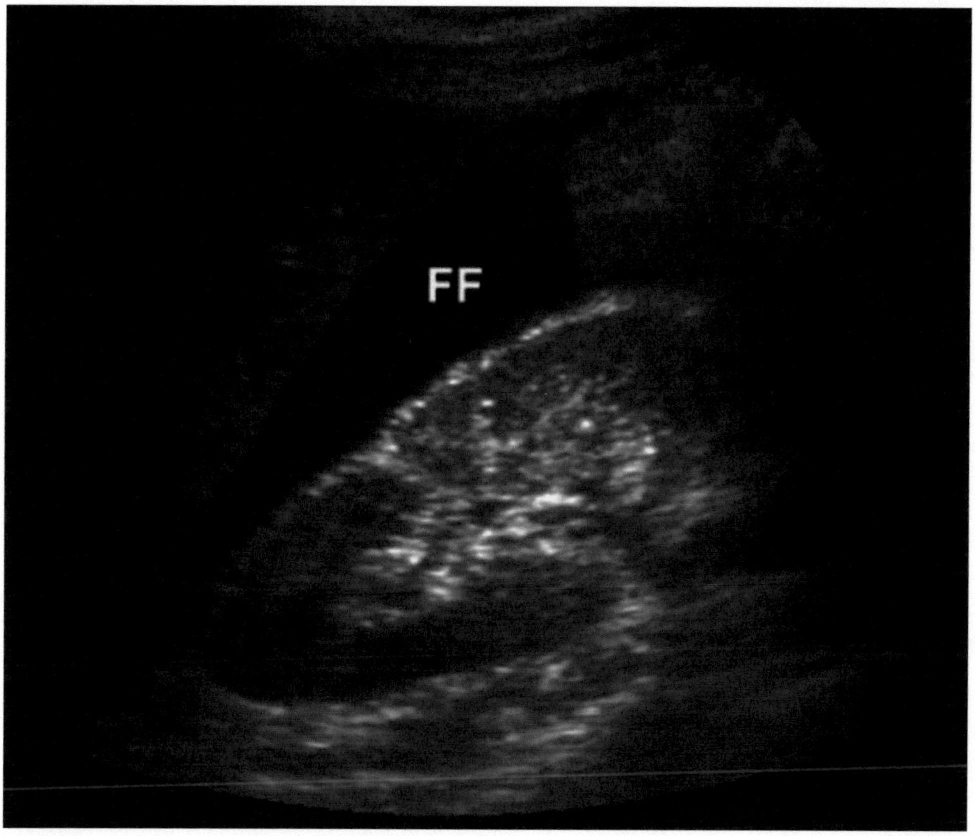

Figure 3.
Ultrasonography demonstrating free fluid adjacent to the kidney, consistent with a large amount of hemoperitoneum in a patient with ruptured ectopic pregnancy.

findings and the diagnosis of ectopic gestation is then based on other sonographic findings like haemoperitoneum, haematosalpinx which present as free fluid in the peritoneal cavity or the pelvis; e.g., in the pouch of Douglas (**Figure 3**). Usually, the identification of an intra-uterine gestation causes shift of attention from the possibility of a concurrent ectopic gestation. Even on suspicion of its existence, identification of ectopic component of heterotopic gestation at ultrasonography is usually much more difficult with the presence of a big haemoperitoneum. In a patient with even a confirmed intra-uterine gestation and presents with acute lower abdominal pain, the likelihood of an ectopic component of a heterotopic gestation must be seriously thought about. Heterotopic gestation is uncommon in natural cycles but it still happen. With the increasing application of assisted reproductive techniques, clinicians must be aware of the fact that identifying an intra-uterine or ectopic gestation clinically or sonographically does not exclude a concurrent existence of ectopic or intrauterine gestation pregnancy, respectively [17, 18].

5. Differential diagnosis

In a patient with an intrauterine pregnancy, the differential diagnosis of uterine bleeding and/or abdominal pain includes threatened abortion, ruptured corpus luteum cyst, and heterotopic pregnancy. The correct diagnosis depends on careful sonographic assessment. Free fluid in the abdomen is a nonspecific finding as it could reflect cyst rupture, tubal pregnancy rupture, or ascites associated with ovarian hyper-stimulation syndrome during ART [16]. Patients with an intrauterine pregnancy may also develop abdominal pain from appendicitis, nephrolithiasis, or urinary tract infection, but these disorders can be distinguished from ectopic pregnancy by history, physical examination, and imaging and laboratory results. In unstable pregnant patients with abdominal pain and bleeding, surgical evaluation continues to play a key role in the diagnosis of heterotopic pregnancies.

6. Treatment

As soon as the diagnosis is made, the extra-uterine pregnancy is always managed surgically especially with features of rupture and the intrauterine component is left to continue normally. With unruptured extra-uterine pregnancy, other treatment options like expectant management with aspiration and installation of potassium chloride or prostaglandin into the ectopic gestational sac can be tried. Methotrexate (MTX) (systemic or local injection) is avoided in heterotopic pregnancy due to its toxicity. Laparoscopic technique is another feasible approach for both cases without disruption to the progression of an intra-uterine pregnancy.

7. Outcome

There appears to be a higher risk of spontaneous abortion of the intrauterine pregnancy of a heterotopic pregnancy than in an isolated intrauterine pregnancy [19]. In a literature review of 11 cases of heterotopic tubal and intrauterine pregnancy treated with Potassium chloride injection, 6 of 11 cases (55%) failed this therapy and required surgical intervention.

8. Conclusion

Clinicians should be aware that the presence of an intra-uterine pregnancy sonographically or clinically should not and does not necessarily exclude the possibility of an ectopic pregnancy which should be thought about in any pregnant patient presents with abdominal pain plus unexplained hypovolemic shock.

9. Summary

Heterotopic pregnancy refers to simultaneous pregnancies at two different implantation sites: an intrauterine and an extra-uterine pregnancy. Heterotopic intrauterine and tubal pregnancies should be suspected when ultrasound examination shows an intrauterine pregnancy and a complex adnexal mass, especially after assisted reproduction technology (ART) is used for conception. The diagnosis is confirmed when the adnexal mass contains a yolk sac or embryo/fetal pole. The clinical presentation closely mimics the symptoms of threatened abortion and isolated ectopic pregnancy. The uterus is enlarged consistent with gestational age and there may be abdominal pain, vaginal bleeding, and/or an adnexal mass. Patients are usually diagnosed late after becoming symptomatic and are often diagnosed at a more advanced gestational age than isolated tubal pregnancy. Rupture can result in acute abdomen and hemodynamic shock. The ectopic pregnancy should be terminated. Treatment of the ectopic pregnancy is tailored to the site of implantation and should utilise the least invasive therapy in order to preserve the concomitant intrauterine pregnancy. Salpingectomy is the standard surgical approach of a coexistent tubal pregnancy and should be the first line of treatment in patients with hemodynamic instability or other signs of tubal rupture. In expert hands, an unruptured ectopic pregnancy can be treated with local feticidal injection under sonographic guidance.

Author details

Bahati Johnson
Obstetrician and Gynaecologist at St. Francis Hospital Mutolere, Kisoro, Southwest Uganda

*Address all correspondence to: johnsonbahati@gmail.com

References

[1] Reece EA et al. Combined intrauterine and extrauterine gestations: A review. American Journal of Obstetrics and Gynecology. 1983;**146**(3):323-330

[2] Govindarajan M, Rajan R. Heterotopic pregnancy in natural conception. Journal of Human Reproductive Sciences. 2008;**1**(1):37

[3] Gruber I et al. Heterotopic pregnancy: Report of three cases. Wiener Klinische Wochenschrift. 2002;**114**(5-6):229-232

[4] Pisarska MD, Carson SA. Incidence and risk factors for ectopic pregnancy. Clinical Obstetrics and Gynecology. 1999;**42**(1):2-8

[5] Luo X et al. Heterotopic pregnancy following in vitro fertilization and embryo transfer: 12 cases report. Archives of Gynecology and Obstetrics. 2009;**280**(2):325-329

[6] Xiao S et al. Study on the incidence and influences on heterotopic pregnancy from embryo transfer of fresh cycles and frozen-thawed cycles. Journal of Assisted Reproduction and Genetics. 2018;**35**(4):677-681

[7] Jerrard D et al. Unsuspected heterotopic pregnancy in a woman without risk factors. The American Journal of Emergency Medicine. 1992;**10**(1):58-60

[8] Barrenetxea G et al. Heterotopic pregnancy: Two cases and a comparative review. Fertility and Sterility. 2007;**87**(2):417

[9] Alsunaidi MI. An unexpected spontaneous triplet heterotopic pregnancy. Saudi Medical Journal. 2005;**26**(1):136-138

[10] Jeong HC et al. Heterotopic triplet pregnancy with bilateral tubal and intrauterine pregnancy after spontaneous conception. European Journal of Obstetrics and Gynecology and Reproductive Biology. 2009;**142**(2):161-162

[11] Varras M et al. Heterotopic pregnancy in a natural conception cycle presenting with tubal rupture: A case report and review of the literature. European Journal of Obstetrics & Gynecology and Reproductive Biology. 2003;**106**(1):79-82

[12] Wallach EE et al. Heterotopic pregnancy after ovulation induction and assisted reproductive technologies: A literature review from 1971 to 1993. Fertility and Sterility. 1996;**66**(1):1-12

[13] Wu Z et al. Clinical analysis of 50 patients with heterotopic pregnancy after ovulation induction or embryo transfer. European Journal of Medical Research. 2018;**23**(1):17

[14] Tandon R et al. Spontaneous heterotopic pregnancy with tubal rupture: A case report and review of the literature. Journal of Medical Case Reports. 2009;**3**(1):1-3

[15] Fleischer A et al. Ectopic pregnancy: Features at transvaginal sonography. Radiology. 1990;**174**(2):375-378

[16] Louis-Sylvestre C et al. The role of laparoscopy in the diagnosis and management of heterotopic pregnancies. Human Reproduction (Oxford, England). 1997;**12**(5):1100-1102

[17] Hassani K et al. Heterotopic pregnancy: A diagnosis we should suspect more often. Journal of Emergency Trauma Shock. 2010;**3**(3):304

[18] Saha E et al. Laparoscopic management of tubal ectopic of heterotopic pregnancy. Journal of Bangladesh College of Physicians and Surgeons. 2016;**34**(4):218-221

[19] Goldstein JS et al. Risk of surgery after use of potassium chloride for treatment of tubal heterotopic pregnancy. Obstetrics & Gynecology. 2006;**107**(2):506-508

Chapter 2

Endoscopic Approach to Ectopic Pregnancy

Sergio Rosales-Ortiz, Tammy Na Shieli Barrón Martínez, Carlos Augusto De La Cruz Vázquez, José Fugarolas Marín, Alejandra Vega León, Janeth Márquez-Acosta, Smarth Santacruz Baez and Rogelio Apolo Aguado Pérez

Abstract

Minimally invasive surgery is an option in the management of ectopic pregnancy, it may be rupture, not rupture, or complement of medical treatment. In addition to the known advantages of endoscopic surgery in the field of obstetrics, it allows better conservative management of the fallopian tube and ovaries, allowing a better reproductive prognosis. The surgical technique to be performed of the clinical findings, the hemodynamic status, and the anatomical location of the ectopic pregnancy. Salpingectomy is performed in the ruptured ectopic pregnancy, assessing the integrity of the contralateral salpinge. Linear salpingostomy is performed on unbroken ectopic pregnancy preserving the fallopian tube, in the literature, this technique has reported maintenance of the fertility rate. In case of a cervical or niche ectopic pregnancy, resectoscopy is recommended.

Keywords: ectopic pregnancy, laparoscopic surgery, hysterocopic procedures

1. Introduction

Ectopic pregnancy occurs in 0.6–2.1% of all pregnancies. Its prevalence in emergency services is 18%, and it is associated with abdominal pain and transvaginal bleeding. It leads to 2.7–5% of maternal deaths in developed countries, and it is also the main cause of death in the first trimester. Death results mainly from ectopic pregnancy rupture. The frequency of ectopic pregnancy is 90–97% in the uterine tube, 1–3% in the ovary, the same percentage is in the niche or cesarean section scar, 1% are abdominal, and 1% are interstitial or located in the horn, as well as cervical, post-hysterectomy, in the rudimentary horn due to Müllerian malformation, and heterotopic or atypical implantation is present in less than 1% of cases. Ectopic pregnancies in atypical locations are a surgical challenge, associated with a high risk of hemorrhage and death, and should be managed in a tertiary care medical center with experience in the treatment of this entity.

Management by laparoscopy and hysteroscopy is currently the most recommended approach; these minimally invasive procedures aid in the preservation of reproductive function, allowing an intrauterine pregnancy within 2 years after conservative surgery in 70% of cases.

2. Endoscopy in gynecology

The implementation of endoscopic surgery in surgical practice is one of the most successful innovations in the history of medicine. The first laparoscopy in a human being was performed by Hans Christian Jacobaeus, who coined the term "laparoscopy," and in 1910 he described the technique to inspect peritoneal, thoracic, and pericardial cavities in humans [1].

Over the following four decades, gynecological laparoscopy was greatly promoted and developed by Raoul Palmer and Hans Frangenheim, who routinely performed the procedure, and the first book on surgical techniques in laparoscopy was published by Patrick Steptoe in 1967. Initially, gynecological laparoscopy was mainly used to establish diagnoses, and its only surgical applications were uterine tubal ligation and fenestration of benign ovarian cysts. Its progressive development, particularly in the last two decades, has placed this surgical technique as the first-line therapeutic approach in gynecological surgery since the same procedures as in open surgery can be performed to manage uterine tubes, ovaries, and corpus uteri pathology; it is also of use in pregnant patients with appendicular, gallbladder, and adnexal disease and in all variants of ectopic pregnancy. It is also the diagnostic and therapeutic gold standard in the management of endometrial pathology [1–6].

Minimally invasive surgery has many advantages in gynecology since it can be performed in girls, adolescents, women of reproductive age, pre and postmenopausal females, including those with obesity; postoperative results include less pain, shorter hospital stays, faster recovery, a decrease in the risk of developing adhesions, a superior esthetic outcome, greater fertility preservation, and the ability of the patient to engage more rapidly in their work and daily activities with less labor disability periods than cases who undergo open surgery. In-office and surgical hysteroscopy is one of the most significant advances in gynecology and has revolutionized the management of intracavitary uterine pathology [7, 8].

Complications of endoscopic surgery in gynecology occur in 3 to 6 cases per 1000 procedures. Half of them appear when introducing the trochars or the hysteroscope, followed by events derived from the use of energy. New entry techniques, materials, and endoscopic equipment have not modified this frequency in the last two decades, but it varies in accordance with the surgical group's experience [1].

3. Endoscopic management of ectopic pregnancy

Surgical management of ectopic pregnancy is the option in patients that are not candidates for expectant or pharmacologic management. The choice between laparoscopy and laparotomy depends on the patient's clinical features, the physician's experience in endoscopic techniques, and the available hospital resources. When possible, an endoscopic approach in the management of this pathology is preferable since there is sufficient evidence of its feasibility and greater preservation of organ function [9–11].

Ectopic pregnancy is specifically managed according to the implantation site that may be: tubal, interstitial, ovarian, abdominal, cervical, or heterotopic.

4. Tubal pregnancy

Ectopic pregnancy in the uterine tube is located in the ampulla in 70–80% of cases, in the fimbriae in 11%, and 10–12% are implanted in the isthmic portion. The intramural or interstitial portion is considered a separate entity [9, 11, 12]. In any of these clinical presentations, women prefer conservative surgical management, and preservation of the uterine tube, despite an increased risk of ectopic pregnancy recurrence, or its persistence [9–11].

According to the ACOG and NICE guidelines, an ectopic pregnancy with a detectable heart rate by ultrasound, an adnexal mass larger than 35 millimeters, a β-hCG fraction of 5000 IU/L, severe abdominal pain, signs and symptoms suggesting ectopic pregnancy rupture, hemodynamic instability, intra-abdominal bleeding, and/or medical treatment failure are all obligate indications of surgery [11].

The laparoscopic surgical techniques in the uterine tube include:

Salpingotomy: This refers to a linear incision on the uterine tube exactly over the ectopic pregnancy on the anti-mesosalpinx border. The uterine tube wall is previously injected with diluted vasopressin (0.2 UI/ml of saline), the longitudinal incision is created with scissors or bipolar energy, and should measure 10–20 millimeters; the embryo and trophoblastic tissue are extracted through the incision by hydrodissection and/or blunt dissection, the surgical site should then be thoroughly washed with anti-adherent solutions, hemostasis should be carefully performed, and the incision closed with absorbable 4/0 sutures [12].

Linear salpingostomy: This is the same procedure as salpingotomy but without suturing the incision.

Salpingectomy: This is the only radical or nonconservative management of the uterine tube and implies the removal of a segment or the entire uterine tube; it is warranted if the uterine tube ruptures, a complication of the previously mentioned techniques, or if further pregnancies are unwanted. This technique may be converted into conservative management if complemented with anastomosis of the uterine tube segments, to preserve function.

Fimbrial milking refers to the nontraumatic compression of the fimbriae to promote trophoblastic expulsion.

Regardless of location, the success of conservative management will be greater if the diagnosis is timely and precedes rupture symptoms [10, 13].

Salpingotomy is recommended in patients wishing to preserve their fertility butare at risk of infertility due to injury in the contralateral tube secondary to pelvic inflammatory disease, or recurrent ectopic pregnancy in the same salpinx; the procedure is feasible in 96% of cases, it is safe, with almost a zero percentage of complications [10]. Its disadvantages include: it requires β-hCG follow-up after surgery to ensure the resolution of the ectopic pregnancy, it carries a greater risk of ectopic pregnancy persistence that may require postoperative treatment in 7% vs. <1% after salpingectomy (RR 15.0; 95% CI 2.0–113.4), and a possible increase in the risk of ectopic recurrence that in the literature, varies between a RR of 2.27 (95% CI 1.12–4.58; $p = 0.02$) to 1.04 (95% CI 0.89–1.21; $p = 0.61$) [9, 14].

Salpingectomy is recommended when there is an extensive injury to the involved salpinx while the contralateral salpinx is intact, and the patient wishes to remain fertile [11]; it carries a lower risk of ectopic persistence, surgical reintervention, and recurrence. Its disadvantage is a decrease in fertility in women with a contralateral injured tube or the presence of pelvic adhesions (40 vs. 75%; $p < 0.005$) [9, 15].

Segmental resection with anastomosis is the recommended procedure in isthmic pregnancy (12% of ectopic pregnancies), since the muscular portion is compact and rapidly invaded by the trophoblast, leading to two significant risks: early rupture and persistence of the trophoblast, as well as sequelae due to structural injury upon removal. This approach requires microsurgical techniques and experienced surgeons [13].

Fimbrial milking or expression is a procedure used in pregnancies implanted in the distal portion of the uterine tube (fimbriae). It is evacuated by compressing the fimbriae with nontraumatic instruments, in the direction of the uterus toward the fimbriae, even with tempered glass atraumatic mobilizers. This technique requires follow-up to exclude the persistence of trophoblastic tissue [10].

In daily practice, the choice between a salpingectomy and a salpingostomy entails patient and physician factors. The patient factors include age, the desire to remain fertile, the obstetric history, previous surgeries, the condition of the involved, and the contralateral tubes. From a medical perspective, the physician's experience in endoscopic surgery and his/her preference, are pivotal.

When conservatively managing the uterine tube, hemorrhage control at the implantation site resulting from the removed tissue is a key, as well as control of post-incision bleeding, for if persistent, a salpingectomy will be required; for this reason, 20% of salpingostomies require conversion into a salpingectomy.

The recommended hemostatic techniques are: direct compression over the surgical site with endoscopic forceps, cauterization with bipolar energy, ligation of the mesosalpinx and bleeding vessels with 6/0 polyglactin, application of hemostatic sealants, and segmental resection with anastomosis of the compromised segment [10, 12].

Direct compression tends to be insufficient while electric energy must be cautiously used to avoid desiccation of the surgical site, since the thermal injury of the mesosalpinx may be permanent and irreversible. If choosing bleeding blood vessel ligation, one must avoid the involvement of the collateral vasculature. Hemostatic sealants must not be used in excess since they may compromise the healing process, and alter the functionality of the tubal epithelium. One must remember that the milder the injury to the tissue, the less formation of adhesions.

When following conservative management, the risk of persistence of trophoblastic tissue may reach 20% but can be decreased with 2% intramuscular prophylactic methotrexate (RR 0.89, 95% CI 0.82, 0.98) [16].

Although there is a tendency to follow conservative management to improve future fertility, no statistical difference has been reported using a particular technique, especially when attempting a subsequent intrauterine pregnancy.

5. Interstitial or horn pregnancy

The terms interstitial pregnancy or horn pregnancy are used indistinctly in the literature to refer to the implantation of the gestational sac in the uterine horns or the proximal portion of the uterine tube (intramural); however, some authors consider that the term "horn pregnancy" should be reserved for gestation in the horn of a bicornuate uterus. The interstitial portion of the uterine tube is that crossing the myometrium to the endometrial cavity; its diameter is 0.7 millimeters and measures 1–2 centimeters in length [17, 18].

The frequency of interstitial pregnancy ranges between 2 and 4% of all ectopic pregnancies, and carries a seven-fold increase in morbimortality compared with other types of tubal pregnancies; this results from the pregnancy's asymptomatic nature until weeks 7 to 16, and that is later suddenly manifested as a massive intraperitoneal hemorrhage, pain, and shock. Its incidence has increased in the past two decades as a result of pelvic inflammatory disease, assisted reproduction techniques, the use of intrauterine devices, adhesions, and previous tubal surgeries [19, 20].

Three therapeutic approaches have been described: close surveillance of the ectopic pregnancy if not associated with hemodynamic instability, medical management, and surgical management. The choice hinges on various factors such as the patient's clinical status, the gestational age at the time of diagnosis, the presence of contraindications of medical treatment, and the patient's preference [21].

An expectant approach (surveillance) is reserved for patients with decreasing β-hCG levels and that remain clinically stable. Medical treatment with local and/or systemic methotrexate is indicated in young nulliparous women wishing to preserve their future fertility if the interstitial pregnancy has not ruptured, if the gestational sac measures 35 mm or more in diameter, a β-hCG level of 5000 mUI/mL or below, and the absence of embryonic cardiac activity; the rate of success is 80% [21–24].

Surgical approaches include: hysteroscopy, laparoscopy, and laparotomy. Surgery is recommended in symptomatic cases that are hemodynamically unstable, and at risk of rupture of the ectopic mass; also, in pregnancies over 7 weeks, gestational sacs ≥35 mm in diameter, when the use of methotrexate is contraindicated or has failed, and according to the patient's preference and the surgeons' expertise [19, 24].

The most frequent approach used to be a laparotomy with horn resection and/or hysterectomy, due to delayed diagnoses, in patients with uterine rupture, hemorrhage, and instability. Currently, this remains an option in the absence of a surgeon with laparoscopic training. Now, the first option is conservative laparoscopy since it is associated with lower blood volume loss, a shorter operative duration, shorter hospital stays, faster recovery, and preservation of the anatomy, even in cases of uterine rupture and hemoperitoneum [23–25].

The endoscopic options are: laparoscopic horn resection, wedge horn resection (in combination with an ipsilateral salpingectomy), hornostomy/salpingostomy (incision in the horn region, and removal of the gestational sac or horn evacuation), and mini-horn excision. The most frequently used and described techniques are laparoscopic horn excision and hornostomy [21, 24, 26].

Less radical techniques that conserve the anatomy such as hornostomy, salpingostomy, and horn mini-excision are performed when the tumor formed by the ectopic implantation of the gestational sac is smaller than 40 millimeters in diameter, there is no rupture nor embryonic cardiac activity, the patient wishes to preserve her future fertility, or the contralateral tube is absent or injured. There is no evidence of subsequent successful pregnancies, but there is a risk of persistent ectopic pregnancy in 5–15% of cases [19, 24].

More radical techniques are preferred such as wedge horn resection with salpingectomy in cases of tumors formed by the ectopic implantation of the gestational sac greater than 40 millimeters in diameter, and in the presence of rupture or embryonic cardiac activity [24]. Between horn resection and laparoscopic hornostomy, there are no significant differences in postoperative hemoglobin level, persistence of the ectopic pregnancy, complications, but only in the duration of surgery, favoring hornostomy [27].

Despite the different laparoscopic techniques, there is no consensus on which is superior, and the most frequent injury is intestinal, due to electrocautery. Vasopressin or a myometrium vasoconstrictor can be injected around the ectopic site to minimize bleeding and obtain hemostasis [24, 28].

There are case reports of hysteroscopic extraction of horn pregnancies, with or without previous methotrexate administration. To evacuate the gestational sac, graspers or forceps are used. Follow-up is based on ultrasound, hysteroscopy, and β-hCG determinations for 3 months [29, 30]. Hysteroscopic management is recommended in horn pregnancies measuring less than 40 millimeters in diameter; if the embryo has no cardiac activity, this approach has greater chances of success with average blood loss of 30 milliliters, but the technique should be limited to groups with expertise in the field [31].

6. Ovarian pregnancy

Ovarian pregnancies account for 0.5–3% of all ectopic processes. Seventy-five percent end in the first trimester and they are often mistaken for a corpus luteum or a tubal ectopic pregnancy by ultrasound.

The clinical presentation is abdominal pain (93%) with scant transvaginal bleeding, and the diagnosis is corroborated at the time of laparoscopy. Management options include wedge resection, sac resection from the ovarian tissue, blunt dissection of trophoblastic tissue (with bipolar energy), and in extreme cases, oophorectomy [9].

Ovarian wedge resection consists in removing the ovarian portion fixed to the ectopic pregnancy; bipolar energy is recommended without suturing the ovarian edges. Hemostasis is obtained with bipolar energy, but in cases of persistent bleeding, an absorbable 2/0 suture should be used.

The gestational sac may be removed from the ovarian surface by hydrosection, or blunt dissection, and complemented with bipolar energy to release trophoblastic tissue or control bleeding on the ovarian surface.

Oophorectomy is reserved for cases in which there is ovarian parenchymal rupture and massive hemorrhage, advanced pregnancies, or a ruptured ectopic pregnancy with infiltration into the ovarian parenchyma.

A laparoscopic approach is recommended over an open technique since it permits greater preservation of the ovarian tissue [11, 32].

7. Abdominal pregnancy

It accounts for 0.1 to 1.3% of all ectopic pregnancies; implantation may occur anywhere in the abdominal cavity, although it is more frequent in the posterior cul-de-sac (approximately 50%), followed by the mesosalpinx (27%). They have also been reported on the omentum, intestine, mesentery, pelvic peritoneum, anterior cul-de-sac, liver, spleen, diaphragm, retroperitoneum, abdominal wall, inferior vena cava, and aorta; however, the entire cavity is at risk of implantation [13, 33].

This type of pregnancy has an eight-fold increased risk of leading to death than tubal pregnancies since it is difficult to diagnose and treat. It is frequently a transoperative finding triggered by clinical signs of an acute abdomen, there is free blood in the abdominal cavity, the presence of an abdominal tumor, or even a fetus associated with an empty uterus on ultrasound.

For study purposes, it can be divided into primary and secondary: primary refers to pregnancies that from the beginning are implanted in the abdominal cavity, while the secondary types are implanted in the abdominal cavity after an extraction procedure or detachment from the site of origin in the genital tract. It has also been divided according to the moment of interruption: early, if it occurs before week 20, or late if the pregnancy culminates after that week [11, 32].

Trophoblastreimplantation after removal of a primary ectopic pregnancy by laparoscopy or laparotomy has a frequency of 1–1.9%. To prevent this, it is important to remove all pathological tissue during surgery as well as clots, to decrease the possibility of leaving reimplantation tissue behind. The Trendelenburg position is recommended as well as the complementary administration of methotrexate [34].

When an early pregnancy is suspected, the recommended treatment is methotrexate, even if the implantation site has not been established; this is followed by laparoscopic excision.

In pregnancies beyond 8–10 weeks of gestation, and at imminent risk of hemorrhage, the decision to perform open or laparoscopic surgery will depend on the time of diagnosis and the patient's clinical status. Manipulation of the placenta and/or placental bed tends to be lethal so the cord must be ligated as close to its insertion as possible and its management should be expectant. The risk of bleeding due to removal must be well evaluated since hemorrhaging of the placental bed results from its location in a tissue that does not contract like the uterus to staunch the bleeding. Within the expectant management, also consider the risk of infection, the possibility of bleeding, and the need for reintervention; the approach should be multidisciplinary [9].

8. Heterotopic pregnancy

It is defined as the simultaneous presence of an intrauterine and an extrauterine pregnancy; it is a very unusual variant with a frequency of approximately 1 in 30,000 spontaneous pregnancies, or 1 in 1111 pregnancies, and tends to result from fertility issues. The most frequent location is the uterine tube but it may also be located in the horn, cervix, niche, or the abdomen [9].

Management of the uterine tube will be the same as in tubal single pregnancy, but salpingectomy is the most frequently reported approach. In other sites, instead of using methotrexate that is contraindicated due to the intrauterine pregnancy, an intracardiac injection of potassium chloride is administered. Management options will depend on the patient's preferences, her clinical conditions, and the physician group's experience. After resolution, the patient requires close follow-up [9, 11].

A complication of laparoscopic treatment is the persistence of trophoblast tissue so β-hCG levels must be followed from day 5 to 10, and if they decrease ≥93.1%, the possibility of persistence is extremely low [35].

9. Cervical pregnancy

Cervical pregnancy has a frequency of 0.1% of all ectopic pregnancies, but its incidence varies from 1 in 1000 to 1 in 18,000 in the literature. Since its etiology is unknown, consider risk factors such as previous dilation and curettage in a previous pregnancy (70% of cases), a previous cesarean section, cervical surgery, and endometritis. Its most common symptom is usually profuse vaginal bleeding, and the diagnostic suspicion should be corroborated by high-resolution ultrasound [36–38].

This type of ectopic pregnancy carries a high risk of massive hemorrhage during abortion labor or during attempts at surgical evacuation; it may even lead to definitive treatment such as an emergency hysterectomy.

Conservative management of the cervical ectopic pregnancy with hysteroscopy was first described in 1996 by Ash and Farrel. It must be performed before the 8th week, there must be no embryonic vitality, and it warrants the use of methotrexate [36, 39, 40].

Hysteroscopic treatment is effective and safe but requires two conditions: if the embryo is alive, the uterine arteries must first be ligated or embolized. If it is alive in an early pregnancy, saline (KCl) or 50% glucose solution or methotrexate can be injected, leading to embryonic death. Once either premise is fulfilled and in accordance with the medical group's experience, hysteroscopy can be performed with local vasopressors and a resectoscope or bipolar miniresectoscope in one or two surgical attempts, with roller ball coagulation [41–44].

With a coagulation intensity of 80 watts and a cut of 60 watts, the implantation site is located and coagulated from the periphery and advanced concentrically until it decreases completely or as far as the implantation site allows blood flow. The cutting and extraction of the gestational sac and trophoblastic tissue can be complemented with Forester's clamp or uterine clamp. Hemostasis is corroborated and supplemented with roller handle selectively. If bleeding occurs, a Foley catheter can be placed, filling the balloon with 5–7 cc of solution and removing it after 7 days.

Postsurgical monitoring should include a determination of β-hCG level every 48 hours until it is negative and a hysterosonography or hysterosalpingography 3 months after the procedure is performed.

10. Niche, cesarean scar pregnancy

This ectopic pregnancy variant is also known as "cesarean" scar, and previously, as isthmocele. The first report of this type of ectopic pregnancy appeared in 1978, and to date, its incidence is 0.15%, with a described frequency of 1 in 1800 to 2216 ectopic pregnancies [45].

It is important to emphasize that the gestational sac may become implanted in a cesarean scar, after a myomectomy, placental removal, or dilation and curettage, even after *in vitro* fertilization.

The diagnosis is difficult to establish whereby the differential diagnoses include cervical ectopic pregnancy and intrauterine pregnancy in abortion labor. Ultrasound findings include the absence of an intrauterine gestational sac, location in the endocervical canal or isthmus surrounded by cesarean scar tissue, with or without myometrium contiguous to the bladder or abdominal cavity; a Doppler image with a gestational sac within the scar defect and surrounded by high-speed vascular flow has also been described.

Niche pregnancies may be divided into two types: type I or endogenic in which the pregnancy grows toward the isthmo-cervical space or uterine cavity, and there is myometrium between it and the bladder; this pregnancy may cause transvaginal bleeding originating in the placental bed. Type II or exogenic invades the bladder or the abdominal cavity, there is no myometrium, and it is usually complicated by uterine rupture and profuse bleeding in an early pregnancy [46].

Before hysteroscopy, 4 milliliters of 50% glucose solution may be injected into the gestational sac, followed by 2.5 mg orally administered methotrexate, 3 times daily for 5 days, or the injection of methotrexate 50 mg/m^2 directly into the gestational sac. Once the embryo's death is corroborated, the niche pregnancy can be removed with a 5Fr resectoscope or a miniresectoscope and bipolar energy, or a mechanical resector (True Clear); note that only type I niche ectopic pregnancies can be treated hysteroscopically [47].

The technique of hysteroscopic surgical resection was mentioned in cervical pregnancy, remembering that if the thickness of the myometrium is less than 3 mm it is dangerous to perform the hysteroscopic technique due to the risk of perforation and bladder injury.

Type II must be treated with an abdominal approach by laparotomy or laparoscopy dissecting or even a vaginal approach. The bladder and resecting uterine and vesical tissue can be performed wit bipolar energy, scalpel, or scissors. The uterus is treated with revival and hemostasis of surgical edges and myography in 2 planes with absorbable 4/0 suture, and a Foley catheter for hemostasis control. Laparoscopy is recommended.

Niche pregnancy can be removed by resectoscopy after the administration of methotrexate, saline solution or ethanol, to provoke embryonic and trophoblastic cell death if there is intercalated myometrium [47].

11. Fertility and ectopic pregnancy

Ectopic pregnancy is a problem with consequences in women of reproductive age, and its resolution requires consideration of the patient's reproductive future. Based on this principle, laparoscopic surgery and hysteroscopy, following the previously described techniques, are part of its conservative management.

The choice of a surgical technique should consider preservation of the patient's life, preservation of the organ and its function, the possibility of persistent trophoblastic tissue or ectopic pregnancy recurrence, the possibility of requiring surgical reintervention, and/or the development of hemorrhage. An important factor to take into account in any conservative management setting is that the contralateral side (uterine and ovarian tubes) must be healthy or without apparent pathology [48].

Other points to consider to preserve the fertility rate with conservative techniques are: the decrease in trophoblastic tissue persistence (5–20%), a single 1 mg/kg intramuscular and/or local dose [49], and an increase in ectopic pregnancy recurrence resulting from the loss of uterine tube function due to scarring, inflammation, and injury caused by bipolar energy during hemostasis, all promoting the implantation of the blastocyst at the scar site [50, 51].

Despite the tendency to follow conservative management protocols, there is no significant difference after a 24–36-month follow-up with either radical treatment or removal of the involved segment, in terms of the frequency of intrauterine pregnancy (HR 1.06 (0.69–1.63; P1/4.78); the recurrence rate is 6–10% [50, 52].

Regardless of whether management is conservative or radical, we must be aware that the spontaneous fertility rate at 2 years is similar as long as there are no risk factors favoring another ectopic pregnancy; if present, radical treatment may certainly compromise spontaneous fertility.

Author details

Sergio Rosales-Ortiz*, Tammy Na Shieli Barrón Martínez,
Carlos Augusto De La Cruz Vázquez, José Fugarolas Marín, Alejandra Vega León,
Janeth Márquez-Acosta, Smarth Santacruz Baez and Rogelio Apolo Aguado Pérez
Hospital de Gineco Obstetricia No. 4 "Luis Castelazo Ayala," Institution
MexicanodelSeguro Social, Mexico City, Mexico

*Address all correspondence to: dr.sergiorosalesortiz@gmail.com

References

[1] Levy L, Tsaltas J. Recent advances in benign gynecological laparoscopic surgery. Faculty Reviewes. 2021;**10**:60

[2] Alkatout I, Mettler L. Hysterectomy a comprehensive surgical approach. In: Histerectomía. Germany: Springer International Publishing; 2018. p. 1676

[3] Hawe JA, Garry R. Histerectomíalaparoscópica. Surgical Innovation. 1999;**6**:80

[4] Ball E, Waters N, Cooper N, Talati C, Mallick R, Rabas S, et al. Evidence-based guideline on laparoscopy in pregnancy: Commissioned by the British Society for Gynaecological Endoscopy (BSGE) Endorsed by the Royal College of Obstetricians and Gynaecologists (RCOG). Facts Views and Vision Obstetrics and Gynaecology. 2019;**11**(1):5

[5] Committee on Practice Bulletins-Gynecology. ACOG practice bulletin 191: Tubal ectopic pregnancy. Obstetrics and Gynecology. 2018;**131**:2, e65

[6] Raznikiewicz A, Korlacki W, Grabowski A. The role of laparoscopy in paediatric and adolescent gynaecology. Miniinvasive Techniques / Wideochirurgia i Inne Techniki Malo Inwazyjne. 2020;**15**(3):424

[7] Stoval DW, Fernandez AS, Cohen SA. Laparoscopy training in United States obstetric and gynecology residency programs. JSLS. 2006;**10**(1):11

[8] Po L, Thomas J, Mills K, Zakhari A, Tulandi T, Shuman M, et al. Guideline No. 414: Management of pregnancy of unknown location and tubal and nontubal ectopic pregnancies. Journal of Obstetrics and Gynaecology Canada. 2021;**43**(5):614

[9] Song T, Lee DH, Kim HC, Seong SJ. Laparoscopic tube-preserving surgical procedures for ectopic tubal pregnancy. Obstetrics Gynecology Science. 2016; **59**(6):512

[10] Tsakiridis I, Giouleka S, Mamopoulos A, Athanasiadis A, Dagklis T. Diagnosis and management of ectopic pregnancy: A comparative review of major national guidelines. Obstetrical & Gynecological Survey. 2020;**75**(10):611

[11] Fujishita A, Masuzaki H, Khan KN, Kitajima M, Hiraki K, Ishimaru T. Laparoscopic salpingotomy for tubal pregnancy: Comparison of linear salpimgotomy with and without suturing. Human Reproduction. 2004;**19**(5):1195

[12] Fylstra DL. Ectopic pregnancy not within the (distal) fallopian tube: Etiology, diagnosis, and treatment. American Journal of Obstetrics and Gynecology. 2012;**206**(4):289

[13] Mol F, Van Mello NM, Strandell A, Strandell K, Jurkovic D, Ross J, et al. European Surgery in Ectopic Pregnancy (ESEP) study group. Salpingotomy versus salpingectomy in women with tubal pregnancy (ESEP study): An open-label, multicentre, randomised controlled trial. Lancet. 2014;**383**(9927):1483

[14] Cheng X, Tian X, Yan Z, Jia M, Deng J, Wang Y, et al. Comparison of the fertility outcome of salpingotomy and salpingectomy in women with tubal pregnancy: A systematic review and meta-analysis. PLoS One. 2016;**11**(3):e0152343

[15] Mol F, Mol BW, Ankum WM, Van der Veen F, Hajenius PJ. Current evidence

on surgery, systemic methotrexate and expectant management in the treatment of tubal ectopic pregnancy: A systematic review and meta-analysis. Human Reproduction Update. 2008;**14**(4):309

[16] Faraj R, Steel M. Management of cornual (interstitial) pregnancy. The Obstetrician and Gynaecologist. 2007;**9**:249

[17] Diagnosis and management of ectopic pregnancy: Green-top Guideline 21. BJOG. 2016;**123**(13):e15

[18] Moawad NS, Mahajan ST, Moniz MH, Taylor SE, Hurd WW. Current diagnosis and treatment of interstitial pregnancy. American Journal of Obstetrics and Gynecology. 2010;**202**(1):15

[19] Soriano D, Vicus D, Mashiach R, Sciff E, Seidman D, Goldenberg M. Laparoscopic treatment of cornual pregnancy: A series of 20 consecutive cases. Fertility and Sterility. 2008; **90**(3):839

[20] Marchand G, Taher Masoud A, Sainz K, Azadi A, Ware K, Vallejo J, et al. A systematic review and meta-analysis of laparotomy compared with laparoscopic management of interstitial pregnancy. Facts Views and Vision Obstetrics and Gynaecology. 2021;**12**(4):299

[21] Marchand G, Masoud AT, Galitsky A, Azadi A, Ware K, Vallejo J, et al. Management of interstitial pregnancy in the era of laparoscopy: A meta-analysis of 855 case studies compared with traditional techniques. Obstetrics Gynecology Science. 2021;**64**(2):156

[22] Lipscomb GH, McCord ML, Stovall TG, Huff G, Portera SG, Ling FW. Predictors of success of methotrexate treatment in women with tubal ectopic pregnancies. The New England Journal of Medicine. 1999;**341**(26):1974

[23] Cucinella G, Calagna G, Rotolo S, Granese R, Saitta S, Tonni G, et al. Interstitial pregnancy: a 'road map' of surgical treatment based on a systematic review of the literature. Gynecologic and Obstetric Investigation. 2014;**78**:141

[24] Afifi Y, Mahmud A, Fatma A. Hemostatic techniques for laparoscopic management of cornual pregnancy: Double-impact devascularization technique. Journal of Minimally Invasive Gynecology. 2016;**23**(2):274

[25] Ng S, Hamontri S, Chua I, Chern B, Siow A. Laparoscopic management of 53 cases of cornual ectopic pregnancy. Fertility and Sterility. 2009;**92**(2):448

[26] Lee MH, Im SY, Kim MK, Shin SY, Park WI. Comparison of laparoscopic cornual resection and cornuotomy for interstitial pregnancy. Journal of Minimally Invasive Gynecology. 2017;**24**(3):397

[27] Bettaiah R, Kamath SS. Intramyometrial injection of vasopressin: A novel method for hemostasis at laparoscopic management of cornual ectopic. Journal of Minimally Invasive Gynecology. 2017;**24**(7):1071

[28] Pal B, Akinfenwa O, Harrington K. Hysteroscopic management of cornual ectopic pregnancy. BJOG. 2003;**110**(9):879

[29] Minelli L, Landi S, Trivella G, Fiaccavento A, Barbieri F. Cornual pregnancy successfully treated by suction curettage and operative hysteroscopy. BJOG. 2003;**110**(12):1132

[30] Kim JS, Nam KH, Lee HH. Hysteroscopic management of cornual pregnancy. Korean Journal of Obstetrics and Gynecology. 2009;**52**(12):1313

[31] Alalade AO, Smith FJE, Kendall CE, Odejinmi F. Evidence-based management

of non-tubal ectopic pregnancies. Journal of Obstetrics and Gynaecology. 2017;**37**(8):982

[32] Atrash HK, Friede A, Hogue CJ. Abdominal pregnancy in the United States: Frequency and maternal mortality. Obstetrics and Gynecology. 1987;**69**(3 Pt 1):333

[33] Schyum AC, Rosendal BB, Andersen B. Peritoneal reimplantation of trophoblastic tissue following laparoscopic treatment of ectopic pregnancy: A case report and review of literature. Journal of Gynecology and Obstetrics Human Reproduction. 2019;**48**(3):213

[34] Ting WH, Lin HH, Hsiao SM. Factors predicting persistent ectopic pregnancy after laparoscopic salpingostomy or salpingotomy for tubal pregnancy: A retrospective cohort study. Journal of Minimally Invasive Gynecology. 2019;**26**(6):1036

[35] Ash S, Farrell SA. Hysteroscopic resection of a cervical ectopic pregnancy. Fertility and Sterility. 1996;**66**(5):842

[36] Tanos V, ElAkhras S, Kaya B. Hysteroscopic management of cervical pregnancy: Case series and review of the literatura. Jurnal of Gynecology Obstetrics Human Reproduction. 2019;**48**(4):247

[37] Matteo M, Nappi L, Rosenberg P, Greco P. Combined medical-hysteroscopic conservative treatment of a viable cervical pregnancy: A case report. Journal of Minimally Invasive Gynecology. 2006;**13**(4):345

[38] Hardy TJ. Hysteroscopic resection of a cervical ectopic pregnancy. The Journal of the American Association of Gynecologic Laparoscopists. 2002;**9**(3):370

[39] Stabile G, Mangino FP, Romano F, Zinicola G, Ricci G. Ectopic cervical pregnancy: Treatment route. Medicina (Kaunas, Lithuania). 2020;**56**(6):293

[40] Mangino FP, Romano F, Di Lorenzo G, Buonomo F, De Santo D, Scrimin F, et al. Total hysteroscopic treatment of cervical pregnancy: "The two steps technique". Journal of Minimally Invasive Gynecology. 2019;**26**(6):1011

[41] Kung FT, Lin H, Hsu TY, Chang CY, Huang HW, Huang LY, et al. Differential diagnosis of suspected cervical pregnancy and conservative treatment with the combination of laparoscopy-asisted uterine artery ligation and hysteroscopicendocervical resection. Fertility and Sterility. 2004;**81**(6):1642

[42] Maglic R, Rakic A, Nikolic B, Maglic D, Jokanovic P, Mihajlovic S. Managementofcervicalectopicpregnancy with small-caliber hysteroscopy. JSLS. 2021;**25**(2):e2021.00016

[43] Di Spiezio SA, Vieira MDC, Lagana AS, Chiofalo B, Vitale SG, Scala M. Combined systemic and hysteroscopic intra-amniotic injection of methrotexate associated with hysteroscopic resection for cervical pregnancy: A cutting-edge approach for an uncommon condition. Eurasian Journal of Medicine. 2017;**49**(1):66

[44] Glenn TL, Bembry J, Findley AD, Yaklic JL, Bhagavath B, Gagneux P, et al. Cesarean scar ectopic pregnancy: Current management strategies. Obstetrical & Gynecological Survey. 2018;**73**(5):293

[45] Gonzalez N, Tulandi T. Cesarean scar pregnancy: A systematic review. Journal of Minimally Invasive Gynecology. 2017;**24**(5):731

[46] Pan Y, Liu MB. The value of hysteroscopic management of cesarean

scar pregnancy: A report of 44 cases. Taiwanese Journal of Obstetrics & Gynecology. 2017;**56**(2):139

[47] Capmas P, Bouyer J, Fernandez H. Treatment of ectopic pregnancies in 2014:new answers to some old questions. Fertility and Sterility. 2014;**101**(3):615

[48] Graczykowski JW, Mishell DR Jr. Methotrexate prophylaxis for persistent ectopic pregnacy after conservativa treatment by salpingostomy. Obstetrics and Gynecology. 1997;**89**(1):118

[49] Chen L, Zhu D, Wu Q, Yu Y. Fertility outcomes after laparoscopic salpingectomy or salpingotomy for tubal ectopic pregnancy: A retrospective cohort study of 95 patients. International Journal of Surgery. 2017;**48**:59

[50] Li J, Jiang K, Zhao F. Fertility outcome analysis after surgical management of tubal ectopic pregnancy: a retrospective cohort study. BMJ Open. 2015;**5**(9):e007339

[51] Fernandez H, Capmas P, Lucot JP, Resch B, Panel P, Bouyer J, et al. Fertility after ectopic pregnancy: The DEMETER randomized trial. Human Reproduction. 2013;**28**(5):1247

[52] Turan V. Fertility outcomes subsequent to treatment of tubal ectopic pregnancy in younger Turkish women. Journal of Pediatric and Adolescent Gynecology. 2011;**24**(5):251

Chapter 3

Medical Management of Ectopic Pregnancy

Maged Shendy, Sonia Abhishek, Lisa Dhege and Ibrahim Alatwi

Abstract

Methotrexate is the standard medical management for ectopic pregnancy. Pharmacologically, it is a folic acid antagonist which inhibits DNA synthesis. 90% of appropriately selected un-ruptured none live ectopic pregnancy respond to methotrexate treatment with no further management is required. In the UK, NICE guidance has identified the selection criteria to achieve the best and safest outcome in ectopic pregnancy treatment with methotrexate. Methotrexate also has a role in management of pregnancy of unknown location. Single administration of 50 mg/m2 body surface area is the most widely acceptable regimen for methotrexate in treatment of ectopic pregnancy. Post treatment b-HCG checks at day 0, 4 and 7 are also a widely accepted follow up regimen to ensure satisfactory decline in b-HCG levels. Methotrexate has a role also in managing none tubal ectopic pregnancies where surgical risks are high. Post treatment transient pain is common and represent a clinical challenge as it can also be failed treatment with ruptured ectopic pregnancy.

Keywords: methotrexate, folic acid antagonist, un-ruptured, none live, single administration, post treatment b-HCG checks

1. Introduction

Single dose of 50 mg/m2 body surface area is the most widely acceptable regimen for methotrexate in treatment of ectopic pregnancy. In carefully selected cases it has comparable success rate to surgical management and avoiding the relevant risks associated with surgical approach [1, 2]. 90% of *appropriately selected* un-ruptured none live ectopic pregnancy respond to methotrexate treatment with no further management is required [3]. Post treatment b-HCG checks at day 1, day 4 and 7 are also a widely accepted follow up regimen to ensure satisfactory decline in b-HCG levels [4].

2. Pharmacology of methotrexate

Methotrexate is a folate antagonist that eneters the cells by active transport process. Once in the cell it becomes polyglutamated and binds dihydrofolate reductase enzyme which subsequently deprive the cell of the folic acid coenzymes. Folic acid co-enzymes are essential for nucleic acid and protein synthesis. Methotrexate suppression of dihydrofolate reductase leads to significant reduction in DNA, RNA and intracellular protein synthesis and ultimately cell death [5]. The most common side effects are nausea, vomiting and diarrhoea. Less commonly it can cause stomatitis, erythema, rash, alopecia and urticaria. Uncommon but serious side effects are also the impacts of its administration on renal and hepatic function. Pretreatment liver and kidney function tests are important as its administration should be carefully weighted with side effects in patients with pre-treatment impaired hepatic and/or kidney functions [5].

3. Selection criteria

Appropriate patient selection is essential for considering the methotrexate in patient with ectopic pregnancy. Appropriate candidate should has; [6–8].

Haemodynamic stability.
Serum b-hCG between under 5000 iu.
No fetal cardiac activity seen on ultrasound scan.
No intrauterine pregnancy.
No significant pain.
Un-ruptured ectopic pregnancy with a mass smaller than 35 mm.
Minimal (under 100 ml) or no free fluid in pouch of Douglas on scan.
No liver, renal impairment.
No bone marrow impairment evidenced by leukopenia, thrombocytopenia or anaemia.

4. Administration

Women who choose this form of treatment should be given written information leaflet and advice about potential of abdominal pain after the treatment and informing to seek medical attention in such situations [9, 10].

Women also should be avoid consuming alcohol, folate containing vitamins and excessive exposure to sun (risk of photosensitive skin reaction) in the post treatment period [11].

Day 1 - FBC check as well as b-hCG, U&Es and Liver function tests. Also women should have blood group and Rh status checked.

Day 4 - symptoms check and b-hCG.

Day 7 - symptoms check and b-hCG, FBC, U&Es and Liver function tests.

Fall of b-hCG levels between day 4 and day 7 should be more than 15% and weekly after day 7 till the b-hCG levels are less than 15 iu.

If less than 15% decrease is reported or levels remains static a second dose of methotrexate should be considered provided a repeat Ultrasound is done exclude fatal cardiac activity and/or appearance of haemoperitonium.

5. Contraindication to methotrexate

Patient who is unstable haemodynamically [12, 13].

Presence of an intrauterine pregnancy.
Breastfeeding.
Previous sensitivity to methotrexate.
Chronic liver disease.
Chronic kidney disease.
Immunodeficiency.
Patient with known bone marrow suppression.

6. Success of methotrexate

With appropriate selection of candidates, methotrexate success can be as high as 91%. There are notable variation across various units in relation to success rates (65–96%) which is especially related the cut off point of b-hCG level for methotrexate consideration.

Approximately 13% requires a second dose of methotrexate with a range of 3–27%.

The most important factors identified for determining the success of the methotrexate treatment includes;

Pre-treatment b-hCG levels; success rate can be as high as 98% with initial levels are under 1000 iu and as low as 38% if the initial levels are over 5000 iu [12].

Pre- treatment ultrasonic findings; presence of fatal pole with cardiac activity is associated with higher failure rate and it is considered a contraindication for methotrexate administration [12–14].

Post - treatment drop in b-hCG; success rates approaches 90% with decrease in b-hCG levels between day 1 and day 4 and between 4 and day 7. This compared to approximate success of 40% if b-hCG levels increase and 60% if the the levels remain static [15, 16].

7. Comparison to expectant management

The use of single dose methotrexate systematically is associated with definite higher success in treatment of ectopic pregnancies compared to expectant management. The expectant management is considered for patients who are asymptomatic and b-hCG under 1500 iu and no free fluid in pouch of Douglas as well as sac under 3 cm in diameter with no metal cardiac activity. Also, the expectant management are considered in asymptomatic patients with pregnancy of unknown location (PUL). Randomised controlled trial concluded a success rate 76% in methotrexate group compared to 59% to expectant management group [17].

8. Comparison to surgical management

Compared to the surgical option in those who meet the selection criteria, Methotrexate associated with lower treatment cost, no hospital admission and no surgical risks. Furthermore, evidence reported no difference in future pregnancy outcomes [18].

9. Post treatment pain

Treatment with methotrexate can be associated with post treatment pain which usually occurs between day 3 and day after its administration. It is mainly due tubal abortion and can stay up to 24 hours. Post treatment pain is a clinical challenge as it cannot distinguished from tubal rupture associated with failed treatment. The consideration for hemodynamic state, full clinical review as well as ultrasound feature defines the next step. Post treatment pain is managed expectantly while tubal rupture requires surgical intervention [19, 20].

10. Post methotrexate anti-D

There are limited evidence to recommend the use of anti-D in those enraptured ectopic pregnancies which meet the selection criteria as likelihood of maternal sensitisation is low. The evidence are strong regarding the use of anti-D with surgical management especially the ruptured cases where the chances of maternal sensitisation to fatal cells can be as high as 25% [21]. In the NICE guidance for management of ectopic pregnancy, the recommendation for anti-D is be used for those undergoing surgical management [22].

11. Role in pregnancy of unknown location (PUL)

The term pregnancy of unknown location is associated with the cases where there is a positive pregnancy test and no evidence of intra- or extrauterine pregnancies. Symptomatic cases requires surgical intervention. However asymptomatic cases represent a clinical challenge as It can be a falling extra or intra uterine pregnancies and resolve spontaneously in approximately 41–69% percent of the cases. Additional 30–37% evolves into visible intrauterine or extrauterine pregnancies. The reminder remains asymptomatic cases where the b-hCG fails to decline and does not evolve into either intrauterine or extrauterine [21]. These cases remains with no visible intrauterine or extrauterine pregnancies (by ultrasound and laparoscopy). Those cases can have the b-hCG sub optimally raising or remains static and are manageable with methotrexate. Regular follow up following methotrexate administration is recommended with b-hCG checks at day 1, day 4, day 7 and weekly after until the b-hCG falls below 15 iu [23, 24].

12. Role of methotrexate in ectopic post surgical management

Persistent trophoblast is identified by failure of b-hCG to decline after surgical treatment. It occurs more frequently in patients who are treated by salpingotomy (8%) compared to (less than 1%) in those treated by salpingectomy [25, 26]. Persistent trophoblast after salpingotomy can be managed expectantly or by administration of methotrexate. Methotrexate use provides higher and consistent success and shorter duration of follow ups in those cases compared to expectant management [25].

13. Role of methotrexate in challenging none-tubal ectopic pregnancies

Methotrexate has defined clear role in none tubal ectopic pregnancies where the surgical management is associated with very high morbidity with higher risk of bleeding and technical challenges. These situations include, scar ectopic, ovarian and abdominal ectopics, cervical ectopic pregnancy and interstitial (cornual) ectopic pregnancies [27–29].

Author details

Maged Shendy[1*], Sonia Abhishek[1], Lisa Dhege[1] and Ibrahim Alatwi[2]

1 North Lincolnshire and Goole NHS Trust, UK

2 Pharmaceutical Care Administration, Tabuk Region, Saudi Arabia

*Address all correspondence to: mego_marmar@yahoo.com

References

[1] Saraj AJ, Wilcox JG, Najmabadi S, Stein SM, Johnson MB, Paulson RJ. Resolution of hormonal markers of ectopic gestation: A randomized trial comparing single-dose intramuscular methotrexate with salpingostomy. Obstetrics and Gynecology. 1998; **92**:989-994

[2] Sowter MC, Farquhar CM, Petrie KJ, Gudex G. A randomised trial comparing single dose systemic methotrexate and laparoscopic surgery for the treatment of unruptured tubal pregnancy. BJOG. 2001;**108**:192-203

[3] Lipscomb GH, Gomez IG, Givens VM, Meyer NL, Bran DF. Yolk sac on transvaginal ultrasound as a prognostic indicator in the treatment of ectopic pregnancy with single-dose methotrexate. American Journal of Obstetrics and Gynecology. 2009; **200**:338.e1-338.e4

[4] Stovall TG, Ling FW, Gray LA. Single-dose methotrexate for treatment of ectopic pregnancy. Obstetrics and Gynecology. 1991;**77**:754-757

[5] Harvey RA. In: Clark MA, Finkel R, Rey JA, editors. Lippincotts Illustrated Pharmacology. 5th ed. USA: Methotrexate; 2012. p. 468

[6] Doubilet PM, Benson CB, Bourne T, Blaivas M. Society of Radiologists in Ultrasound Multispecialty Panel on Early First Trimester Diagnosis of Miscarriage and Exclusion of a Viable Intrauterine Pregnancy. Diagnostic criteria for nonviable pregnancy early in the first trimester. The New England Journal of Medicine. 2013;**369**:1443-1451

[7] Bourne T, Barnhart K, Benson CB, Brosens J, Van Calster B, Condous G, et al. NICE guidance on ectopic pregnancy and miscarriage restricts access and choice and may be clinically unsafe. BMJ. 2013;**346**:f197

[8] Craig LB, Khan S. Expectant management of ectopic pregnancy. Clinical Obstetrics and Gynecology. 2012;**55**:461-470

[9] Warren WB, Timor-Tritsch I, Peisner DB, Raju S, Rosen MG. Dating the early pregnancy by sequential appearance of embryonic structures. American Journal of Obstetrics and Gynecology. 1989;**161**:747-753

[10] Timor-Tritsch IE, Farine D, Rosen MC. A close look at early embryonic development with the high frequency transvaginal transducer. American Journal of Obstetrics and Gynecology. 1988;**159**:676-681

[11] Britten S, Soenksen DM, Bustillo M, Coulam CB. Very early (24-56 days from last menstrual period) embryonic heart rate in normal pregnancies. Human Reproduction. 1994;**9**:2424-2426

[12] Kirk E, Condous G, Bourne T. The non-surgical management of ectopic pregnancy. Ultrasound in Obstetrics & Gynecology. 2006;**27**:91-100

[13] Lipscomb GH, Gomez IG, Givens VM, Meyer NL, Bran DF. Yolk sac on transvaginal ultrasound as a prognostic indicator in the treatment of ectopic pregnancy with single-dose methotrexate. American Journal of Obstetrics and Gynecology. 2009; **200**:338.e1-338.e4

[14] Dudley PS, Heard MJ, Sangi-Haghpeykar H, Carson SA, Buster JE. Characterizing ectopic pregnancies

that rupture despite treatment with methotrexate. Fertility and Sterility. 2004;**82**:1374-1378

[15] Trio D, Strobelt N, Picciolo C, Lapinski RH, Ghidini A. Prognostic factors for successful expectant management of ectopic pregnancy. Fertility and Sterility. 1995;**63**:469-472

[16] Nguyen Q, Kapitz M, Downes K, Silva C. Are early human chorionic gonadotropin levels after methotrexate therapy a predictor of response in ectopic pregnancy? American Journal of Obstetrics and Gynecology. 2010;**202**:630.e1-630.e5

[17] van Mello NM, Mol F, Verhoeve HR, van Wely M, Adriaanse AH, Boss EA, et al. Methotrexate or expectant management in women with an ectopic pregnancy or pregnancy of unknown location and low serum hCG concentrations? A randomized comparison. Human Reproduction. 2013;**28**:60-67

[18] Mol B, Hajenius P, Engelsbel S, Ankum W, Hemrika D, Van der Veen F, et al. Treatment of tubal pregnancy in The Netherlands: An economic comparison of systemic methotrexate administration and laparoscopic salpingostomy. American Journal of Obstetrics and Gynecology. 1999;**181**(4):945-951

[19] National Institute for Health and Care Excellence. Ectopic pregnancy and miscarriage. diagnosis and initial management in early pregnancy of ectopic pregnancy and miscarriage. Manchester: NICE: NICE Clinical Guideline 154; 2012

[20] Dudley PS, Heard MJ, Sangi-Haghpeykar H, Carson SA, Buster JE. Characterizing ectopic pregnancies that rupture despite treatment with methotrexate. Fertility and Sterility. 2004;**82**:1374-1378

[21] Hartwell EA. Use of Rh immune globulin: ASCP practice parameter. American Society of Clinical Pathologists. American Journal Clinical Pathology 1998;110:281-292.

[22] Qureshi H, Massey E, Kirwan D, Davies T, Robson S, White J, et al. British Society for Haematology. BCSH guideline for the use of anti-D immunoglobulin for the prevention of haemolytic disease of the fetus and newborn. Transfusion Medicine. 2014;**24**:8-20

[23] Condous G, Okaro E, Khalid A, Zhou Y, Lu C, Van Huffel S, et al. Role of biochemical and ultrasonographic indices in the management of pregnancies of unknown location. Ultrasound in Obstetrics Gynaecology. 2002;**20**(Suppl. 1):36-37

[24] Bourne T, Barnhart K, Benson CB, Brosens J, Van Calster B, Condous G, et al. NICE guidance on ectopic pregnancy and miscarriage restricts access and choice and may be clinically unsafe. BMJ. 2013;**346**:f197

[25] Mol F, van Mello NM, Strandell A, Strandell K, Jurkovic D, Ross J, et al. European Surgery in Ectopic Pregnancy (ESEP) study group. Salpingotomy versus salpingectomy in women with tubal pregnancy (ESEP study): An open-label, multicentre, randomised controlled trial. Lancet. 2014;**383**:1483-1489

[26] Hajenius PJ, Mol BW, Ankum WM, van der Veen F, Bossuyt PM, Lammes FB. Clearance curves of serum human chorionic gonadotrophin for the diagnosis of persistent trophoblast. Human Reproduction. 1995;**10**:683-687

[27] Poole A, Haas D, Magann EF. Early abdominal ectopic pregnancies:

A systematic review of the literature. Gynecologic and Obstetric Investigation. 2012;**74**:249-260

[28] Cassik P, Ofili-Yebovi D, Yazbek J, Lee C, Elson J, Jurkovic D. Factors influencing the success of conservative treatment of interstitial pregnancy. Ultrasound in Obstetrics & Gynecology. 2005;**26**:279-282

[29] Zosmer N, Fuller J, Shaikh H, Johns J, Ross JA. Natural history of early first-trimester pregnancies implanted in Cesarean scars. Ultrasound in Obstetrics & Gynecology. 2015;**46**:367-375

Chapter 4

Diagnosis of Ectopic Pregnancy

Subrat Panda, Ananya Das, Kaushiki Singh, Prateeti Baruah and Anusuya Sharma

Abstract

Ectopic pregnancy is defined as the implantation of a fertilised egg outside the uterine cavity. The site of ectopic pregnancy are Fallopian tube. Cervix, ovary, peritoneal cavity, or uterine scars. Other two site of implantation are cornual pregnancy and interstitial pregnancy. Diagnostic tests for ectopic pregnancy include a urine pregnancy tests, Serum beta hcG and ultrasound. The instant result of a urine pregnancy test is a useful pointer for the clinician to suspect an ectopic pregnancy. The test is a useful triage tool for clinicians to rule out a pregnancy when the clinical situation is not clear such as a patient who is not sure of dates, does not remember or is in a state of shock and the history cannot be elicited. Ultrasound remains the mainstay of the diagnosis and high index of suspicion and a detailed history are pre-requisite of scanning. Different ultrasonography feature are diagnostic of different site of implantation. For uterine scar pregnancy ultrasonologic criteria are not validated still now.

Keywords: ultrasound, b HCG

1. Introduction

The proverb black cat in dark night fits into the diagnosis of ectopic pregnancy. To diagnose ectopic pregnancy clinician's mind should be suspicious about ectopic pregnancy. The most common ectopic site of implantation (97%) is the fallopian tube. The most common site for tubal pregnancy is ampulla, followed by isthmus, fimbrial and interstitial. Sometimes twin tubal pregnancy with both embryos in one tube or with one in each tube has been noted [1]. The other sites of ectopic pregnancies are implantation in the cervix, ovary, peritoneal cavity, or uterine scars. A growing ectopic pregnancy in any location can make the tissue vascular, friable and eventually rupture and result in intra-abdominal bleeding. This is a life threatening medical emergency. In history the risk factors like Pelvic inflammatory disease, including pelvic tuberculosis, previous ectopic pregnancy, pregnancy with an intrauterine device, tubal surgeries (ligations, reconstructions, and re-implantations), history of STD, smoking, infertility, ovulation induction and ART procedures should be elicited. The majority of women with ectopic gestation have no identifiable risk factor.

Ectopic pregnancy should be suspected in any woman with child bearing age presenting to the clinic or emergency department with symptoms of amenorrhea, pain abdomen, and vaginal bleeding [2]. They may present with the complaint of fainting, collapse, breathlessness, or dizziness. Uncommon symptoms include diarrhoea, pain in the shoulder, rectal pressure, urinary symptoms, and anaemia. A small, undisturbed tubal pregnancy, the physical examination might be normal. In these situations, the diagnosis is dependent on investigations. On the other hand, with late presentations, there could be a disturbance of the vital signs and features of shock may be present including tachycardia, tachypnoea, hypotension, and rarely bradycardia. On abdominal examination there may be guarding, rigidity and tenderness. There could be also cervical motion tenderness, adnexal tenderness or fullness in the adnexae and pouch of Douglas. The presence of abdominal signs with altered vital parameters suggests presence of hemoperitoneum and mandates urgent resuscitation and management at a centre with appropriate facilities for blood transfusion and surgery.

Diagnostic tools for ectopic pregnancy are urine pregnancy tests, Serum beta-hCG and transvaginal or trans-abdominal ultrasound. Clinical suspicion combined with these tests plays a very important role in diagnosis and management of ectopic pregnancy. The instant result of a urine pregnancy test is a useful pointer for the practitioner to suspect an ectopic pregnancy. This kit test is easily available at low cost and is reliable. The test is a useful triage tool for clinicians to rule out a pregnancy when the clinical situation is doubtful such as a patient who is not sure of dates, does not remember or is in a state of shock and the history cannot be elicited.

Laboratory tests of a single laboratory value of beta-hCG might not be useful to diagnose the location of a pregnancy. The typical level in a healthy intrauterine pregnancy on the day of the missed period is 50 to 100 IU/L. In a normal intrauterine pregnancy, levels of serum beta-hCG will double every 1.4 to 2.1 days and peak between 50,000 and 100,000 IU/L at 8 to 10 weeks of pregnancy. Compared to the pattern observed in healthy intrauterine pregnancies, the rate of increase between two serum-hCG levels when it is done 48 hours apart is slower.

Progesterone levels are not useful for the diagnosis of an ectopic and maybe used in the prognostication of pregnancy of unknown location.

Ultrasound remains the mainstay of the diagnosis [3]. High index of suspicion and a detailed history are pre-requisite of scanning. The majority of tubal ectopic pregnancies should be visualised on transvaginal ultrasound.

Transvaginal ultrasound has sensitivities of 87.0–99.0% and specificities of 94.0–99.9% for the diagnosis of ectopic pregnancy [4]. Usually most of the ectopic pregnancies will be visualised on the initial ultrasound examination [5]. When no intrauterine or extauterine pregnancy is seen in USG it is called pregnancy of unknown location (PUL). Ectopic pregnancies initially classified as a PUL on the initial scan may be ectopic pregnancies are just too small and too early in the disease process to be visualised on the initial ultrasound examination. Sometimes the limiting value of beta-hCG should be evaluated, below which intrauterine pregnancies cannot be seen on USG. In case of PUL serial beta-hCG level assays adone to identify pattern that indicate either a growing or failing IUP. Without clear evidence for ectopic pregnancy, serial β-hCG level is advised and a level is checked after 48 hours. This wards off unnecessary medical therapy and avoids harming an early normal pregnancy. With more concern for an ectopic gestation, D&C is another option to distinguish an ectopic from a failing IUP. Normal rise B-Hcg does not exclude normal and ectopic pregnancy [6]. Laparoscopy is no longer the gold standard for diagnosis of ectopic pregnancies.

2. USG findings

An inhomogeneous or non cystic adnexal mass is the most common finding, about 50–60% of cases.

An empty extra-uterine gestational sac will be present in around 20–40% [7] of cases and an extra-uterine gestational sac containing a yolk sac and/or embryonic pole that may or may not have cardiac activity will be present in around 15–20% of cases [7].

There is no specific endometrial appearance or thickness, based on which diagnosis of tubal pregnancy can be confirmed. A few of cases, in around 20%, a collection of fluid may be seen within the uterine cavity, known as 'pseudosac'. It is difficult to differentiate pseudosac from an early intrauterine gestational sac. The intradecidual and double decidual signs indicates early intrauterine pregnancy (**Figures 1** and **2**). The intradecidual sign is eccentrically located echogenic area within a markedly thickened decidua [8]. The double decidual sign is described as an intrauterine fluid collection surrounded by two hyper echogenic rings [9]. But practically, it is very difficult to distinguish a 'pseudosac' which is just a collection of fluid in the endometrial cavity from

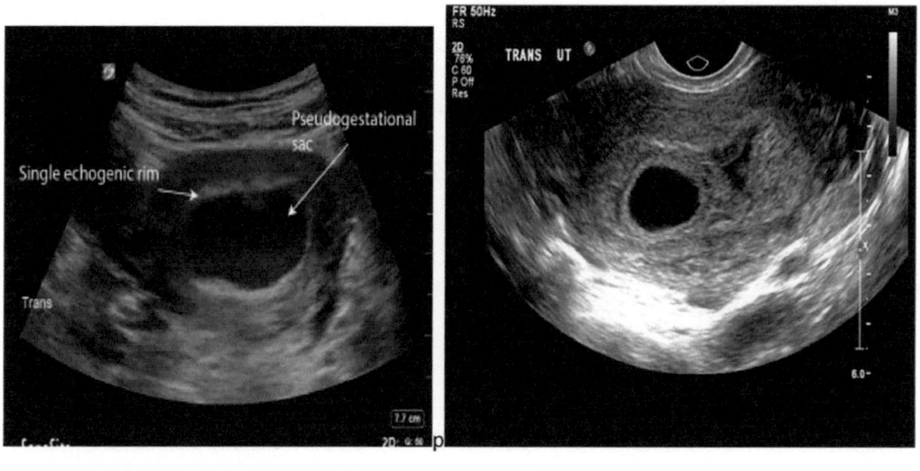

Figure 1.
Double decidual sign.

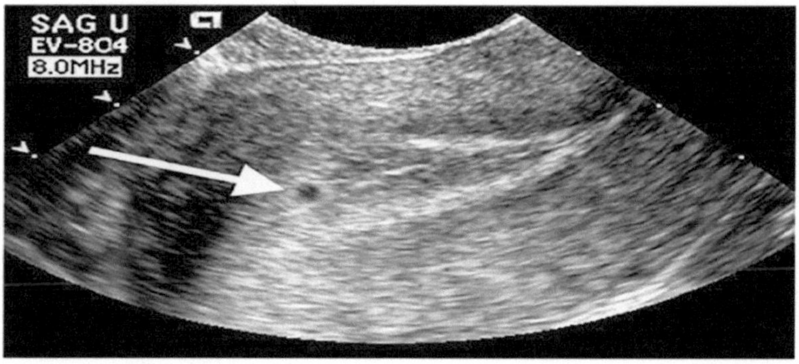

Figure 2.
Intradecidual sign.

an early intrauterine sac. A small anechoic cystic structure is more likely to be an early sac rather than a 'pseudosac'. Positive pregnancy test with and a small anechoic cystic structure without adnexal mass has probability of ectopic pregnancy is 0.02% [9].

When free fluid is seen on ultrasound, it is not a pinpointing feature of ectopic pregnancy. A small amount of anechoic fluid in the pouch of Douglas may be found physiologically in normal pregnancy and may be seen with ectopic pregnancies. Which may signify tubal rupture, Most commonly the echogenic fluid has been reported is due to blood leaking from the fimbrial end of the fallopian tube but it may be tubal rupture. Culdocentesis was used in the past to diagnose hemoperitoneum. Fluid with old blood clots and blood does not clot points to hemoperitoneum. If the blood sample clots it may have been drawn from nearby blood vessel or from profound bleeding ectopic pregnancy. Nowadays culdocentesis is not advised it is replaced by usg.

3. Cervical pregnancy

Cervical ectopic pregnancy is diagnosed by following usg criteria:

1. Empty Uterus

2. a barrel-shaped cervix,

3. a gestational sac is seen below the level of the internal cervical Os,

4. 'Sliding sign' usually absent

5. On colour Doppler, Blood flow around the gestational sac

The 'sliding sign' distinguishes cervical ectopic pregnancies and miscarriages that are within the cervical canal. It is present in cervical miscarriage but absent in cervical ectopic gestation.

When pressure is applied to the cervix using the probe, in a miscarriage, the gestational sac slides against the endocervical canal, but does not in an cervical ectopic gestation.

Cervical Ectopic Gestation usually develops in fibrous wall of the cervix. Risk factors includes previous dilatation and curettage operation and pregnancy due to ART may be implanted in cervical canal [10, 11]. Usually the women present with painless vaginal bleeding and sometimes with massive haemorrhage [12].

Clinical criteria for diagnosis of cervical pregnancy [13].

- Pregnancy with painless vaginal bleeding.

- Soft and expanded cervix with length is equal or more than fundus wasp like or hourglass shape.

- Product of conception firmly attached to cervical canal.

- Closed internal os and partially opened external os (**Figure 3**).

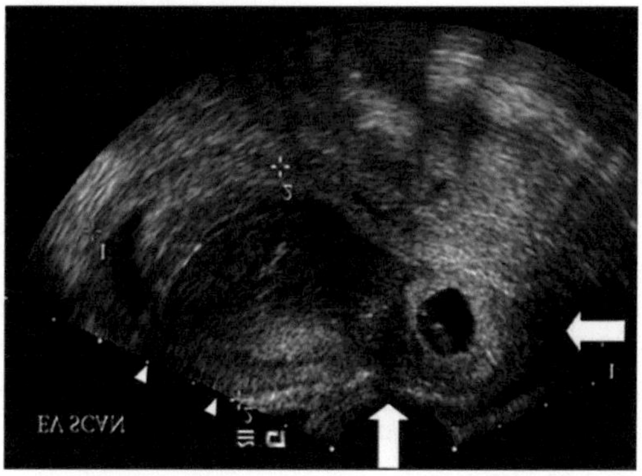

Figure 3.
Cervical pregnancy.

4. Caesarean scar pregnancy

The diagnosis of Caesarean scar pregnancy made by using transvaginal usg sometimes supplemented by trans-abdominal imaging if required.

Magnetic resonance imaging (MRI) can be used as a second-line investigation if the diagnosis is suspicious. Usually women with CSP present with painful bleeding PV and nearly half of women are asymptomatic.

Caesarean scar pregnancy is defined as implantation into the myometrial defect occurring at the site of the previous uterine scar.

The diagnostic criteria described for caesarean scar implantation on transvaginal ultrasound include: [14].

1. Empty uterine cavity and endocervical canal

2. Gestational sac or solid mass of trophoblast located anteriorly at the level of the internal Os embedded at the site of the previous lower uterine segment caesarean section scar

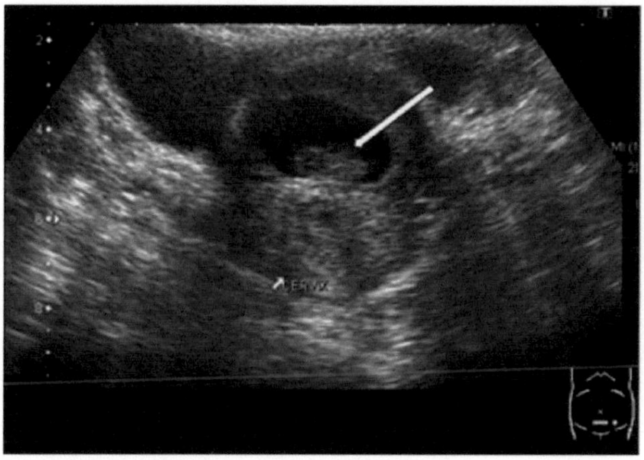

Figure 4.
Caesarean scar pregnancy.

3. Myometrial layer between bladder and gestational sac is absent or thin.

4. Evidence of prominent trophoblastic/placental circulation on Doppler examination.

5. Pregnancy less than 8wks triangular gestational sac is seen previous caesarean scar defect but after 8 weeks of gestation the gestational sac become rounded or oval.

The true prevalence of caesarean scar pregnancies is likely to be somewhat higher than estimated in the literature as some cases end in the first trimester, either by miscarriage or termination, and go unrecorded. A few percentages of reported cases of caesarean scar pregnancy were wrongly diagnosed as intrauterine or cervical pregnancies at presentation (**Figure 4**).

5. Interstitial pregnancy

When the implantation occurs in the proximal part of fallopian tube that lies within the muscular layer of uterus. Ipsilateral salpingectomy is a risk factor for interstitial pregnancy.

The following ultrasound scan criteria may be used for the diagnosis of interstitial pregnancy:

1. Empty uterine cavity, eccentric implantation,>1 cm away from the most lateral edge of uterine cavity.

2. Gestational sac surrounded by less than 5 mm of myometrium in all imaging planes,

3. And presence of the 'interstitial line sign'. An echogenic line extends from gestational sac to uterine cavity. It is highly sensitive and specific.

Dimensional ultrasound may be used if available to avoid misdiagnosis.

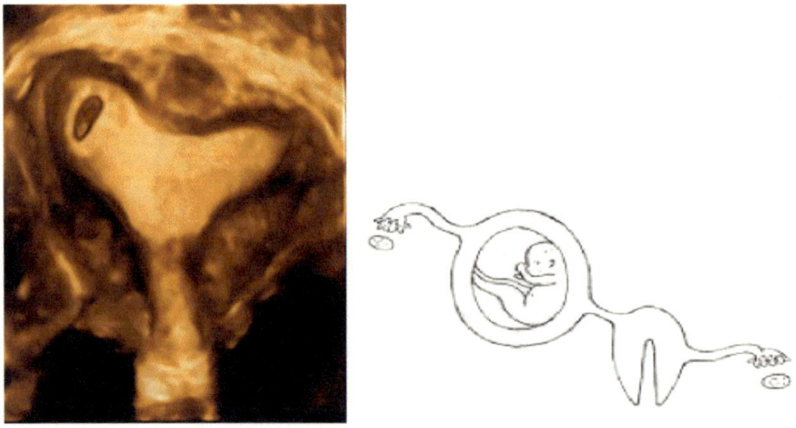

Figure 5.
Interstitial pregnancy.

MRI may be useful in addition to ultrasonography in the diagnosis of interstitial pregnancy (**Figure 5**).

6. Cornual pregnancy

The implantation occurs in the rudimentary horn of uterus it may be communicating or non communicating. It is a confusing terminology. Some authors prefer the cornual pregnancy when implantation occurs in upper lateral part of uterine cavity of normal uterus.

Ultrasound scan criteria are used for the diagnosis of cornual pregnancy:

1. Visualisation of a single interstitial portion of fallopian tube in the main uterine body,

2. gestational sac/products of conception seen mobile and separate from the uterus and completely surrounded by myometrium,

3. And a vascular pedicle adjoining the gestational sac to the unicornuate uterus.

7. Ovarian pregnancy

Findings suggestive of an ovarian ectopic pregnancy on transvaginal ultrasound with an empty uterus are:

1. A wide echogenic ring with an internal anechoic area on the ovary is seen commonly. A yolk sac or embryo is rarely seen [15].

2. It is not possible to separate the cystic structure or gestational sac from the ovary on gentle palpation (negative sliding organ sign).

3. Corpus luteum is identified separately from the suspected ovarian pregnancy.

4. Colour Doppler might be useful to detect foetal heart pulsation within the ovary.

A complex echogenic adnexal mass with free fluid in the pouch of Douglas may be the ruptured ovarian ectopic pregnancy.

Usually it is difficult to distinguish ovarian ectopic pregnancies from corpus luteal cysts, tubal ectopic pregnancy stuck to the ovary, a second corpus luteum, ovarian germ cell tumours and other ovarian pathologies and the diagnosis is confirmed surgically and histologically in most of the cases.

8. Abdominal pregnancy

When the implantation occurs in intraperitoneal cavity excluding tubal,ovarian and intraligamentous pregnancy. Usually the women have vague symptoms or no symptoms. Abnormal foetal position may be palpated.

MRI might be a useful diagnostic adjunct in advanced abdominal pregnancy and can help to plan the surgical approach.

1. Early abdominal Pregnancy, no intrauterine gestational sac.

2. Tubes and ovary are normal

3. A gestational sac surrounded by loops of bowel and separated from them by peritoneum and there is no myometrium between anterior abdominal wall and gestational sac.

4. A wide mobility similar to fluctuation of the sac, particularly evident with pressure of the transvaginal probe toward the posterior cul-de-sac.

Sonographic diagnosis may not be useful. MRI is very much useful to confirm the diagnosis and to identify placental implantation because placenta may be implanted over vital structures, such as major blood vessels and bowel [16]. This can help to make preoperative preparedness for perioperative considerations, such as the surgical approach, requirement of blood products, preoperative angiographic embolisation, bowel preparation and insertion of ureteral catheters. Precise mapping of the location of the placenta by using ultrasound and/or MRI prior to laparotomy to avoid incising the placenta and the associated risk of uncontrollable haemorrhage is necessary.

9. Heterotopic pregnancy

When there are both intrauterine and extrauterine implantation it is called heterotropic gestation it can be diagnosed with ultrasonography.

Heterotopic pregnancy should be suspected in if conception is after assisted reproductive technologies, with an intrauterine pregnancy and complaining of persistent pelvic pain and in those.

women with a persistently raised beta-hCG level following miscarriage or termination of pregnancy. A higher than expected level of serum beta-hCG in relation to gestational age may be suspicious of heterotopic pregnancy but, the presence of a complete or partial mole must be ruled out. Two corpora lutea found on laparoscopy or laparotomy. Sometimes patient may present with hemoperitoeum after termination of normal pregnancy or persistence of enlarged uterus and amenorrhoea after excision of ectopic pregnancy.

10. Conclusion

Ectopic pregnancy is associated with high maternal mortality and morbidity. With early diagnosis complications can be avoided. Primary modality of diagnosis is Ultrasound Scan. Hence Obstetrician should be well trained to diagnose ectopic pregnancy, and clinician should have high index of suspicion to diagnose ectopic pregnancy.

Author details

Subrat Panda*, Ananya Das, Kaushiki Singh, Prateeti Baruah and Anusuya Sharma
NEIGRIHMS, Shillong, Meghalaya, India

Address all correspondence to: pandadrsubrat@rediffmail.com

References

[1] Della-Giustina D, Denny M. Ectopic pregnancy. Emergency Medicine Clinics of North America. 2003;**21**:565-584

[2] Gurel S, Sarikaya B, Gurel K, Akata D. Role of sonography in the diagnosis of ectopic pregnancy. Journal of Clinical Ultrasound. 2007;**35**:509-517

[3] Kirk E, Papageorghiou AT, Condous G, Tan L, Bora S, Bourne T. The diagnostic effectiveness of an initial transvaginal scan indetecting ectopic pregnancy. Human Reproduction. 2007;**22**:2824-2828

[4] Condous G, Van Calster B, Kirk E, Haider Z, Timmerman D, Van Huffel S, et al. Prediction of ectopic pregnancy in women with a pregnancy of unknown location. Ultrasound in Obstetrics & Gynecology. 2007;**29**:680-687

[5] Condous G, Okaro E, Khalid A, Lu C, Van Huffel S, Timmerman D, et al. The accuracy of transvaginal ultrasonography for thediagnosis of ectopic pregnancy prior to surgery. Human Reproduction. 2005;**20**:1404-1409

[6] Shepherd RW, Patton PE, Novy MJ, Burry KA. Serial beta-hCG measurements in the early detection of ectopic pregnancy. Obstetrics and Gynecology. 1990;**75**:417

[7] Yeh HC, Goodman JD, Carr L, Rabinowitz JG. Intradecidual sign: A US criterion of early intrauterine pregnancy. Radiology. 1986;**161**:463-467

[8] Bradley WG, Fiske CE, Filly RA. The double sac sign of early intrauterine pregnancy: Use in exclusion of ectopic pregnancy. Radiology. 1982;**143**:223-226

[9] Doubilet PM, Benson CB. Double sac sign and intradecidual sign in early pregnancy: Interobserver reliability and frequency of occurrence. Journal of Ultrasound in Medicine. 2013;**32**:1207-1214

[10] Ginsburg ES, Frates MC, Rein MS, Fox JH, Hornstein MD, Friedman AJ. Early diagnosis and treatment of cervical pregnancy in an in vitro fertilization program. Fertility and Sterility. 1994;**61**: 966

[11] Jeng CJ, Ko ML, Shen J. Transvaginal ultrasound-guided treatment of cervical pregnancy. Obstetrics & Gynecology. 2007;**109**:1076

[12] Ushakov FB, Elchalal U, Aceman PJ, Schenker JG. Cervical pregnancy: Past and future. Obstetrical & Gynecological Survey. 1997;**52**:45

[13] Paalman R, McElin T. Cervical pregnancy. American Journal of Obstetrics and Gynecology. 1959;**77**:126

[14] Timor-Tritsch IE, Monteagudo A, Santos R, Tsymbal T, Pineda G, Arslan AA. The diagnosis, treatment and follow-up of cesarean scar pregnancy. American Journal of Obstetrics and Gynecology. 2012;**207**:44e1

[15] Comstock C, Huston K, Lee W. The ultrasonographic appearanceof ovarian ectopic pregnancies. Obstetrics & Gynecology. 2005;**105**:42-45

[16] Aliyu LD, Ashimi AO. A multicentre study of advanced abdominal pregnancy: A review of six cases in low resource settings. European Journal of Obstetrics & Gynecology and Reproductive Biology. 2013;**170**:33-38

Chapter 5

Ectopic Pregnancy after Ipsilateral Salpingectomy

Afaf Felemban, Haya Aljurayfani, Fatimah Alamri, Jawaher Alsahabi, Ghadeer L. Aljahdali, Hadeel Alkheelb, Hessa Alkharif and Mohmmad Albugnah

Abstract

Ectopic pregnancy is a significant health problem for women prevalence is increase in patient with history of previous ectopic pregnancy or pelvic surgeries or pelvic inflammatory disease, and widespread treatment with assisted reproductive technologies the incidence of ectopic pregnancies has greatly increased during the past two decades and it is now estimated to occur in 2% of all pregnancies recurrent ectopic pregnancy in the remnant portion of the tube after ipsilateral salpingectomy has only rarely been reported. We present unusual cases of ipsilateral ectopic pregnancy occurring in the stump of a previous ectopic site.

Keywords: ectpoic pregnancy, salpingectomy, tubal stump

1. Introduction

Ectopic pregnancy (EP) is the implantation of a fertilized ovum anywhere outside of the uterine cavity [1].

Ectopic pregnancy still accounts for 4–10% of pregnancy-related deaths and leads to a high incidence of ectopic site gestations in subsequent pregnancies [2]. Early intervention saves lives and reduces morbidity around 90% of ectopic pregnancies occur in one of the fallopian tubes rare sites as in the cervix, ovary, cesarean section scar defect and the abdominal cavity [2, 3].

The fallopian tubes length about 8–10 cm extend from the uterine cornus. The sites of tubal implantation in descending order of frequency are; ampulla (73.3%), isthmus (12.5%), fimbrial (11.6%), and interstitial (2.6%) [4]. If a woman with a previous ectopic gets pregnant, the risk of a recurrent EP is increased four-fold [5].

Recently, literature review reported rare cases of recurrent ectopic pregnancy in the remnant portion of the tube after a previous ipsilateral salpingectomy [6]. Ipsilateral recurrent ectopic pregnancy may occur in the proximal or distal remnant of the operated tube [7, 8].

Ectopic pregnancy in the remnant tube is difficult to diagnose due to the unique anatomic location of the pregnancy sometimes results in delayed diagnosis [6]. Although complete tubal resection cannot prevent cornual pregnancy, it might reduce the risk of recurrent ectopic pregnancy in the remnant tube [6] while the exact incidence of ectopic pregnancy occurred in the remnant tube after ipsilateral adnexectomy is not known [6].

Tubal pregnancy associated with high risk of rupture and severe bleeding [9], due to the poor ability of this portion of the tube to distend as well as the increased vascularity of the area (anastomosis of the uterine and ovarian vessels) [10].

2. Pathophysiology

The mechanism of recurrent ipsilateral ectopic pregnancy is not clear. But there is many hypotheses including contralateral transmigrate of fertilized ovum from the intact fallopian tube across the endometrial cavity to contralateral tubal stump. And another hypotheses transperitoneal migration of the egg or embryo to the contralateral tubal stump or passage of the spermatozoa to fertilize the ovum in the proximal tubal remnant with some degree of patency or recanalization may occur in the tubal stump [6].

Another explanation for the anatomical location of the ectopic pregnancy may be through transperitoneal migration of an ovum from the contralateral ovary to the opposite tube via the pouch of Douglas. This was explained previously, that embryo or ovum migration has been described animals [11]. These findings suggest that normal tubo-ovarian integrity is not essential for pregnancy to occur. The possible paths that the gametes or the fertilized ovum can travel are illustrated in **Figure 1**.

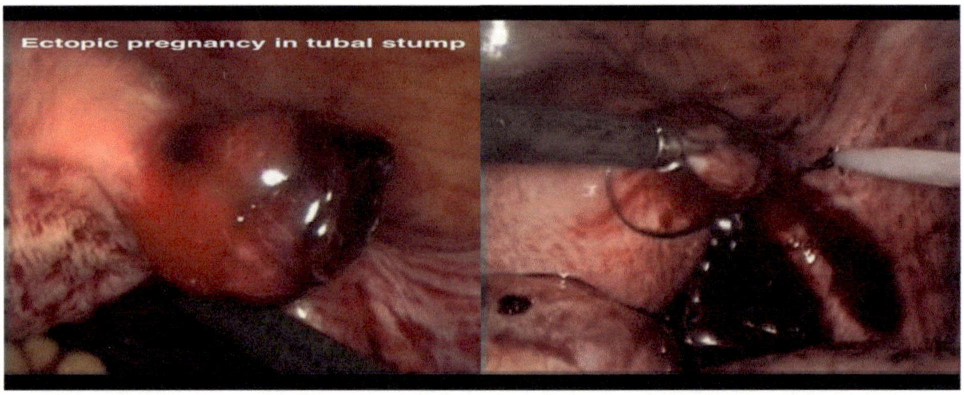

Figure 1.
Laparoscopic appearance of rupture ectopic pregnancy in the proximal remnant of the right Fallopian tube.

A rare case of transperitoneal ovum migration resulting in an intra-uterine pregnancy is presented. A woman with left congenital ovarian absence and a surgically removed right oviduct, conceived following microsurgical repair of left tubal occlusion [12].

3. Diagnosis

Ultrasonographic examination is effective for the diagnosis of tubal stump pregnancy. However, in some cases, the diagnosis of tubal stump pregnancy is difficult because the tubal stump portion is near the ovary (**Figure 2**).

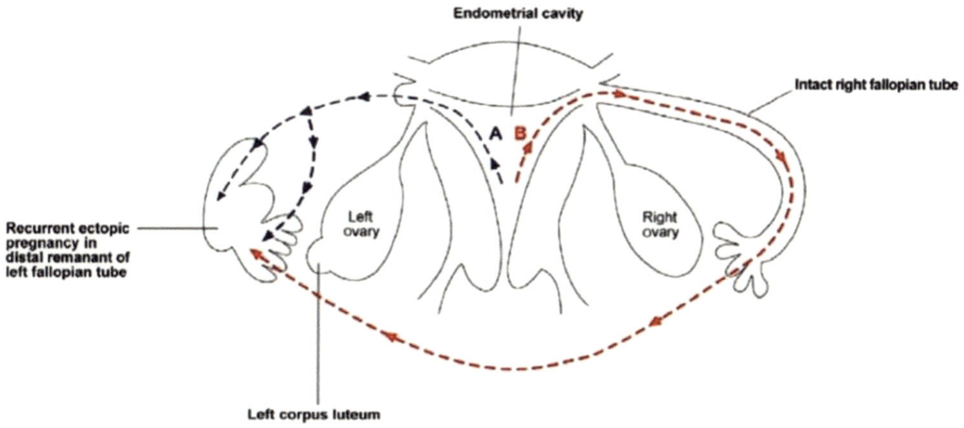

Figure 2.
Proposed hypothesis for reurrect ectopic pregnancy post isplitaeral salpingectomy A: recanalization in the tubal stump B: contralatera transmigrate of fertilized ovum from the intact fallopian tube across the endometrial cavity to contralateral tubal stump.

Ectopic pregnancy occurring in tubal stump after tubectomy is extremely rare, and the frequency of tubal stump pregnancy is approximately 0.4% of all pregnancies [13].

Due to unique anatomic location of the tubal stump pregnancy sometimes results in delayed diagnosis and it will carry high risk of rupture of the uterus in some case increase beyond 12 weeks of amenorrhea, and the rupture of the ectopic part occurs in 20% of ectopic pregnancies beyond 12 weeks of gestational age. Earlier diagnosis would decrease morbidity and increase the chance of successful minimal invasive surgery [13].

The ovarian corpus luteum is mistaken for a tubal stump pregnancy. Moreover, it is thought that many doctors pay less attention to the tube in which patients have already undergone salpingectomy because of ectopic pregnancy.

three sonographic criteria for interstitial and tubal stump pregnancies proposed by Lau and Tulandi:

1. clean uterine cavity (no sac)

2. a gestational sac seen separately and > 1 cm from the most lateral edge of the uterine cavity.

3. with thin myometrial layer surrounding the chorionic sac.7 Using the separameters, they found that the diagnosis was relatively specific (88–93%), but on the other hand, the sensitivity was only 40% for the diagnosis of interstitial and tubal stump pregnancies [13].

Another authors Timor-Tritsch et al., advocate an "interstitial line sign" the diagnosis of interstitial and tubal stump pregnancies [11].

In small-sized interstitial pregnancies, the line may represent the interstitial lesion of the tube. In large-sized interstitial pregnancies, it likely represents the endometrial canal. This sign represents the visualization of an echogenic line extending into the abutting interstitial ectopic mass of the tubal mid-portion. The diagnosis of interstitial pregnancy is 80% sensitive and 98% specific with the "interstitial line sign" technique [13]. Spontaneous interstitial pregnancy on a tubal stump after unilateral salpingectomy followed by vaginal Doppler ultrasound [14].

Per-vaginal color and angio Doppler blood flow analysis combined with serial measurement of human chorionic gonadotrophin (HCG) level is reported here for the first time to study the local vascularity of a cornual pregnancy and to monitor the effectiveness of medical therapy. They found, a strong relationship between morphological changes of trophoblastic tissue and the intensity of neovascularization was noted. Methotrexate (MTX) therapy as systemic single-dose allowed successful treatment of an interstitial ectopic pregnancy involving part of the proximal portion of a tubal stump. Conventional transvaginal ultrasonography Compound color Doppler, the outpatient surveillance of ectopic pregnancy evolution following MTX therapy is greatly enhanced. This is of particular value in cornual pregnancies which are highly likely to develop harmful complications during surgical intervention or even during puncture for local MTX injection [15].

4. Treatment

Lau and Tulandi reported, The main treatment for tubal stump pregnancy is surgery and conservative management using methotrexate that the overall success rates in surgical treatment reached 100% and that of methotrexate management was 83% [16].

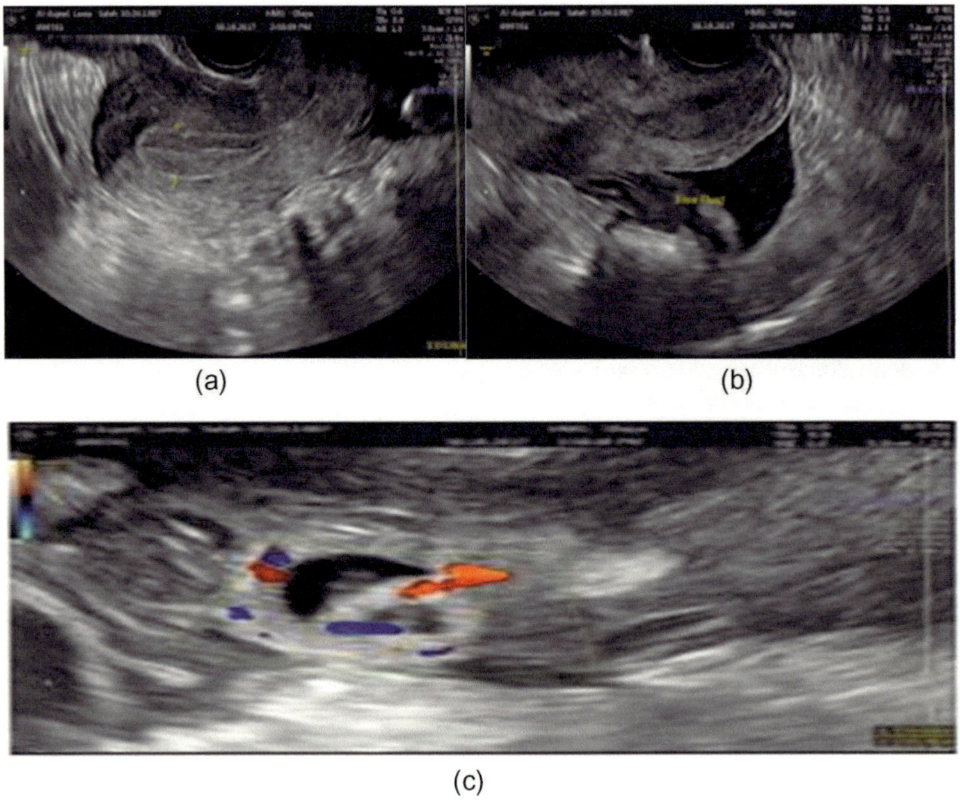

Figure 3.
Sonographic appearance: (A) absence of an intrauterine pregnancy (B) free fluid in the cul de sac (C) a twin ectopic pregnancy in the right adnexa.

The difficulty level of laparoscopic operation for interstitial and tubal stump pregnancy is higher than that of common laparoscopic salpingectomy. The operation method for tubal stump pregnancy is almost the same as that of interstitial pregnancy, and hence, the selection of operative method depends on the surgeon's preference and expertise (**Figure 3**).

There is a lot of successful laparoscopic surgery for interstitial and tubal stump pregnancy using an advanced bipolar device and injecting diluted vasopressin into the uterus [2, 7, 8]. Sherer et al. before incising the cornua, he recommend clamping the adjacent uterine wall to the interstitial pregnancy with long-jaw forceps [17]. Some authors, they are reports of using hysteroscopic surgery for interstitial and tubal stump ectopic pregnancy [12]. However, long-term prognosis for selecting hysteroscopic surgery are unknown.

Any subsequent pregnancy after operation for tubal stump pregnancy should be followed up carefully and cesarean delivery at term may be safer and help decrease the risks of uterine rupture during labor.

In summary, Laparoscopic surgery can be account first-line treatment for a hemodynamically stable patient with interstitial pregnancy of a small size. Sometimes, the accurate diagnosis for this type of ectopic pregnancy is difficult; therefore, we have to pay much attention to the possibility of tubal stump pregnancy when we diagnose the ectopic pregnancy [13, 18].

5. Prevention

There is no certain nature of the mechanism, selecting a method for prevention is difficult. However, there is some options may be suggested to decrease the probability of recurrence of ipsilateral ectopic pregnancy. When performing the tubectomy, care should be taken not to leave a long stump [16] and this remnant portion should be minimized. Additionally, using diathermy or ligation with clips of the proximal portion may be necessary components to decrease the risk of recurrent implantation [9].

Another author, suggest performing hysterosalpingography to evaluate the patency of the fallopian tubes after salpingectomy and ligation [19]. In addition to salpingectomy, he suggests insertion of flexible microinserts (commercial products are available) into the remnant tube. These devices are considered to be effective in occluding the fallopian tubes [11] This can be provided if greater protection left from proximal tube.

In case of the woman has completed her family and has a history of ectopic pregnancy, effective contraception counseling may be given, or permanent contraceptive measures implemented [9].

Clinicians should be aware that one ectopic is a risk factor for future ectopic and that salpingectomy does not exclude ipsilateral ectopic pregnancy.

Ectopic pregnancy on the ipsilateral tube is rare, but we should be aware that history of salpingectomy is a risk factor for future ectopic pregnancy in ipsilateral remnant tube.

6. Discussion

Recurrent ectopic pregnancy in the remnant portion of the tube after ipsilateral salpingectomy has only rarely been reported, The exact incidence of ectopic

Author	Years	History	GA	Diagnosis	Management
Felemban [23]	2017	A29years old G4P1	5 weeks	The right ectopic pregnancy in tubal stump	Systemic single-dose Methotrexate .
Cynthia [24]	2015	A 27 year-old G5P1	NA	Ectopic pregnancy in right tubal remnant .	Resected by laparoscopy
Longoria [25]	2014	A 44-year-old G5P1	8 weeks	**A live twin ectopic pregnancy**	Laparoscopic the remnant of the tube with ectopic pregnancy was resected .
Masakazu [2]	2014	A 26 year-old G4P1	NA	Tubal Stump Pregnancy	Laparoscopic surgery for tubal Stump Pregnancy resection was performed
Bahareh [26]	2013	A 35-year-old G8P2	49 days	Ruptured left ectopic pregnancy	Laparoscopic intervention demonstrated a ruptured left ectopic pregnancy
Bahareh [26]	2013	A42 year-old G11P7	NA	Ectopic pregnancy in the remnant of the right tube.	Laparoscopic resection of the remnant of the right tube.
Sonia [8]	2010	a 35 year-old multiparous	6 weeks	Ectopic pregnancy within the right tube.	Laparoscopy Right salpingectomy and removal of ectopic was performed
Yung-Liang [27]	2009	A 28 year-old G1P0	NA	Ectopic pregnancy in left tube.	Removal of the gestational products and resection of the proximal left fallopian tube were performed laparoscopically.
Tomone Yano [11]	2009	A 35 year-old G7P3	NA	Ectopic pregnancy in the isthmic portion of the left remnant tube.	Laparoscopy tubal stump resected
Tomone Yano [11]	2009	A 34 year-old G1P0	NA	Ectopic pregnancy in right remnant tube.	Laparoscopy excision of tubal stump.
Li-Ling Chou [28]	2008	A 23 year-old G1P0	NA	An ectopic pregnancy in the distal remnant of the right tube	Laparoscopy excision of The distal remnant and the products of conception .
Takeda et al. [6]	2006	A 27 year-old G3P2	6 weeks	Ruptured ectopic pregnancy occurring in the remnant tube	Laparoscopic surgery, ruptured remnant tube was excised.

Author	Years	History	GA	Diagnosis	Management
Takeda et al. [6]	2006	A 36 year-old G2P1	8 weeks	Ectopic pregnancy in the remnant tube	Laparoscopic surgery, the unruptured remnant tube was excised.
Bernardini [10]	1998	A 36 year-old G4P0	52 days	Ectopic pregnancy in the left tubal stump	Systemic single-dose Methotrexate

Table 1.
The results of a literature review of previously reported cases with a history of the previous salpingectomy which diagnosed as a case of ectopic pregnancy in ipsilateral remnant tube with spontaneous conception.

Author	Years	History	Specific history	Diagnosis	Management
Tsuyoshi ota [12]	2016	A 40 years G2P1	History of right salpingectomy	Ectopic pregnancy in right tube stump.	Laparoscopy, tubal stump removed .
Turab [29]	2013	A 33-years G1P0	history of a right salpingectomy	Recurrent ruptured ectopic pregnancy	Laparoscopy was performed, tube stump was resecte with the products of conception

Table 2.
The reported cases of ectopic pregnancy in the remnant tube after ipsilateral salpingectomy induced by ovulation induction intrauterine insemination.

pregnancy occurred in the remnant tube after ipsilateral adnexectomy is not known, Ko et al. reported that tubal stump pregnancy after salpingectomy is extremely rare, with a prevalence of about 0.4% [20]. Takeda et al. reported an incidence of 1.16% in their department from January 1994 to August 2005 [21], with mortality 10–15 times higher compared to other forms of ectopic [22].

Table 1 shows the results of a literature review of previously reported cases with a history of previous salpingectomy which were diagnosed as a ectopic pregnancy in ipsilateral remnant tube with spontaneous conception.

Table 2 shows findings associated with reported cases of ectopic pregnancy in the remnant tube after ipsilateral salpingectomy induced by ovulation induction and intrauterine insemination. Agarwal et al. [30], these authors reported seven cornual and tubal stump pregnancies in patients with prior salpingectomy undergoing IVF. Also, two literature reported cases of ectopic pregnancy in the remnant tube after ipsilateral salpingectomy conceived after IVF, [20] he report Six cases of tubal stump pregnancy, four of six conceived with IVF and all managed surgically, Only one of the cases managed successfully by methotrexate and the remaining six were treated surgically.

The mechanism of recurrent ipsilateral ectopic pregnancy is not clear. But there is many hypotheses including Transperitoneal migration of the egg or embryo to the contralateral tubal stump or Passage of the spermatozoa to fertilize the ovum in the proximal tubal remnant with some degree of patency or recanalization may occur in the tubal stump or contralateral fertilization occurred and the fertilized ovum transmigrate from the intact fallopian tube across the endometrial cavity to contralateral tubal stump.

In The literature review, there are some of the suggestions to decrease the risk of recurrence of ectopic pregnancy in a remnant tube after tubectomy, the length of the remnant tube should be minimized and adequate closer to the tip of the remnant tube achieved by diathermy or using clip.

Author details

Afaf Felemban[1]*, Haya Aljurayfani[1], Fatimah Alamri[1], Jawaher Alsahabi[1], Ghadeer L. Aljahdali[1], Hadeel Alkheelb[1], Hessa Alkharif[1] and Mohmmad Albugnah[2]

1 King Abdulaziz Medical City, Riyadh, Saudi Arabia

2 Dr. Suliman Alhabeb Hospital, Riyadh, Saudi Arabia

*Address all correspondence to: fillimbana@ngha.med.sa

References

[1] Available from: https://www.sciencedirect.com/sdfe/pdf/download/eid/3-s2.0-B9780323032476100115/first-page-pdf

[2] Available from: https://journals.lww.com/clinicalobgyn/Abstract/2012/06000/Ectopic_Pregnancy__History,_Incidence,.3.aspx

[3] Available from: https://academic.oup.com/humupd/article/16/4/432/801230?login=true

[4] Available from: https://onlinelibrary.wiley.com/doi/full/10.1002/j.2205-0140.2010.tb00162.x

[5] Available from: https://d1wqtxts1xzle7.cloudfront.net/65827367/s0020-7292_2802_2900134-020210228-813-58kwu7.pdf?1614561405=&response-content-disposition=inline%3B+filename%3DThree_consecutive_ipsilateral_tubal_preg.pdf&Expires=1634983096&Signature=PgCg~57V2DtDLkC0kVu6SyFGyr50-eaLbjmeNBhQoaJyID48sV-fWUmxX-4m2qjuXYUfD4i8aOij6mcUwka9NrDuz6qm7l8oFHteVkF0tatoblRQTdtx7ENT34fI0Zc7gt-imVe4wssmhk5bjOS5xrkHCL4vtx6a9aVntWIKZ7A6vVXAcZ9AXVZUkDVQzJdjBmHgmFaF8dlyZHR6kd7dpV8RAgG1lptHOZ1h-j74dQ7qxk8r64MczBivx8DlLgTBn34xqpMeQi8tz-awwqFqv3DWhWS9-aYPfQndPdeR5gNQaUs2ZGuOxHJw0b3DkcczbnPjxmOJuXqqahPajS082A__&Key-Pair-Id=APKAJLOHF5GGSLRBV4ZA

[6] Available from: https://www.sciencedirect.com/science/article/pii/S1110569018300086

[7] Available from: https://www.sciencedirect.com/science/article/pii/S1028455913001836

[8] Available from: https://core.ac.uk/download/pdf/82823612.pdf

[9] Available from: https://www.hindawi.com/journals/criog/2013/753269/

[10] Available from: https://obgyn.onlinelibrary.wiley.com/doi/abs/10.1111/j.1447-0756.2

[11] Available from: https://www.birpublications.org/doi/full/10.1259/bjr/95330860

[12] Available from: https://obgyn.onlinelibrary.wiley.com/doi/abs/10.3109/00016348809004285

[13] Available from: https://journals.sagepub.com/doi/full/10.4137/CCRep.S20907

[14] Available from: https://www.ncbi.nlm.nih.gov/pmc/articles/PMC6113952/

[15] Available from: https://academic.oup.com/humrep/article/13/6/1723/815851?login=true

[16] Available from: https://onlinelibrary.wiley.com/doi/full/10.1007/s12522-009-0028-7

[17] Available from: https://europepmc.org/article/med/4019146

[18] Available from: http://www.smj.org.sg/sites/default/files/4609/4609cr1.pdf

[19] Shah V, Panay N, Williamson R, Hemingway A. Hysterosalpingogram: An essential examination following essure hysteroscopic sterilisation. British Journal of Radiology. 2011;**84**(1005):805-812. DOI: 10.1259/bjr/95330860

[20] Ko PC, Liang CC, Lo TS, Huang HY. Six cases of tubal stump pregnancy:

Complication of assisted reproductive technology. Fertility and Sterility. 2011;**95**(7):2432, e1-4. DOI: 10.1016/j.fertnstert.2011.03.069. PMID: 21497804. [Epub 2011 Apr 17]

[21] Takeda A, Manabe S, Mitsui T, Nakamura H. Spontaneous ectopic pregnancy occurring in the isthmic portion of the remnant tube after ipsilateral adnexectomy: Report of two cases. The Journal of Obstetrics and Gynaecology Research. 2006;**32**(2):190-194. DOI: 10.1111/j.1447-0756.2006.00385.x

[22] Samiei-Sarir B, Diehm C. Recurrent ectopic pregnancy in the tubal remnant after salpingectomy. In: Takeuchi K, Usta IM, Badawy SZA, editors. Case Reports in Obstetrics and Gynecology. [Internet]. 2013;**2013**:753269. DOI: 10.1155/2013/753269

[23] Felemban A, Alamri F, Al Bugnah M, Felimban Y, Alkheleb A. Twin ectopic pregnancy after ipsilateral salpingectomy: A report of cases. Middle East Fertility Society Journal. 2018

[24] Available from: https://www.sciencedirect.com/science/article/pii/S2210261214004635

[25] Available from: https://www.sciencedirect.com/science/article/abs/pii/S0015028299002423

[26] Available from: https://search.informit.org/doi/abs/10.3316/INFORMIT.361467677241977

[27] Available from: https://core.ac.uk/download/pdf/82769076.pdf

[28] Available from: https://www.sciencedirect.com/science/article/pii/S1028455908600819

[29] Available from: https://europepmc.org/article/med/8495783

[30] Agarwal SK, Wisot AL, Garzo G, Meldrum DR. Cornual pregnancies in patients with prior salpingectomy undergoing in-vitro fertilization (IVF) and embryo transfer. Fertility and Sterility. 1996;**65**(3):659-660. DOI: 10.1016/s0015-0282(16)58171-0. PMID: 8774304

Section 2

Fetal Malformation

Chapter 6

Prenatal Diagnosis of Diaphragmatic Hernia

Marina Sica, Carlotta Plessi and Francesco Molinaro

Abstract

Congenital diaphragmatic hernia (CDH) is a condition characterized by a defect in the diaphragm leading to protrusion of abdominal contents into the thoracic cavity interfering with normal development of the lungs. The pathophysiology of CDH is a combination of lung hypoplasia and immaturity associated with persistent pulmonary hypertension of newborn (PPHN) and cardiac dysfunction. Prenatal assessment of lung to head ratio (LHR) and position of the liver by ultrasound are used to diagnose and predict outcomes. However, fetal therapy is indicated in cases where negative prognostic factors are detected in screening investigations (liver herniation, LHR <1.0). Immediate management at birth includes bowel decompression, avoidance of mask ventilation and endotracheal tube placement if required. The main focus of management includes gentle ventilation, hemodynamic monitoring and treatment of pulmonary hypertension followed by surgery. Although inhaled nitric oxide is not approved by FDA for the treatment of PPHN induced by CDH. Surgical treatment of CDH should be planned in election, after the achievement of hemodynamic stability. The only case in which it is acceptable to perform an emergency operation is when there are signs of ischemia of the herniated intestinal loops. Extracorporeal membrane oxygenation (ECMO) is typically considered after failure of conventional medical management for infants ≥ 34 weeks' gestation or with weight > 2 kg with CDH and no associated major lethal anomalies. Prematurity, associated abnormalities, severity of PPHN, type of repair and need for ECMO can affect the survival of an infant with CDH. With advances in the management of CDH, the overall survival has improved.

Keywords: lung hypoplasia, pulmonary hypertension, extracorporeal membrane oxygenation, prenatal diagnosis

1. Introduction

Congenital diaphragmatic hernia (CDH) is a congenital malformation of diaphragm, which leads to a defect in separation between the thoracic and abdominal cavities [1, 2]. It appears to be due to an error in the development of the pleuro-peritoneal canals and therefore develops around 6 weeks of gestation [1]. Its incidence is 1:3000 live births. Progress in the management of these patients has significantly increased survival rates (up to 90% [3]), but disease-related morbidity remains very high: the main problem is the compression exerted by the herniated viscera on the developing lungs, development, which causes pulmonary hypoplasia and hypertension [4].

2. Classification

CDH can be classified, depending on the location of the defect, into postero-lateral, or Bochdalek's hernia (70–75%), anterior or Morgagni's hernia (23–28%) and central or hiatal hernia (2–7%) [4]. Morgagni's hernia is often discovered incidentally in older children, as it rarely causes such a mass effect on the thoracic level as to compromise the development of the lungs. Bochdalek's hernia is the form that is classically referred to when talking about this pathology and to which we will refer accordingly in the next paragraphs (26). Most often it is located on the left side (85%), but it can also be right (13%) or bilateral (2%) [4].

3. Pathogenesis

The pathogenesis of CDH is complex and currently still little known. Some studies have shown that pulmonary hypoplasia in these patients arises before the development of the diaphragm itself. This discovery opened the door to the so-called "double hit theory" which sees pulmonary hypoplasia as the result of two insults: the first, affecting both lungs, would be due to genetic and environmental factors (for example alcohol, smoking, obesity, low intake of retinoids during pregnancy); the second, which would affect only the lung ipsilateral to the defect, would consist of the compressive effect of the herniated viscera and their interference with normal fetal respiratory movements. Multiple studies have demonstrated the importance of the genetic component in the pathogenesis of ECD: they often fall within syndromic pictures, and about 40% of cases are associated with other congenital anomalies, especially cardiovascular (11–15% of ECD) [4].

4. Antenatal management

Given the potential severity of the disease, prenatal counseling represents a fundamental phase of the diagnostic-therapeutic process of CDH: parents must be adequately informed about all the steps to be taken and the risks in terms of mortality and morbidity.

4.1 Antenatal diagnosis

Ultrasound currently represents the gold standard in CDH diagnosis, although it has been calculated that less than two-thirds of CDHs are detected on prenatal screening ultrasound scans. The mean gestational age at diagnosis is 24–25 weeks, more advanced in cases of isolated defects than in CDHs associated with other anomalies. The typical ultrasound sign is the presence of abdominal organs (intestinal loops, stomach, liver) in the chest. Indirect signs of CDH can be changes in the heart axis, polyhydramnios, mediastinal shift. The differential diagnosis includes all congenital pulmonary malformations, bronchial atresia, intestinal duplications and mediastinal masses [5, 6]. The execution of genetic tests and second-level imaging tests is essential for defining the prenatal management strategy, whether it is inclined towards termination of pregnancy, or whether it is oriented towards fetal therapies. One of the main prognostic factors is represented by the lung to head ratio (LHR), which by measuring the length of the lung contralateral to the hernia normalized for the head circumference, provides an indirect estimate of pulmonary hypoplasia. More specifically, since the LHR changes with advancing gestational age, we prefer to use the ratio between observed LHR and expected LHR (observed/expected LHR or o/and LHR).

One or/and LHR <25% is indicative of severe hypoplasia, while one/and LHR of 25–35% or an LHR of 35–45% with herniated liver are indicative of moderate hypoplasia. In fact, another prognostic factor is represented by the position of the liver: since the liver and the fetal lung are poorly distinguishable ultrasonographically, there may be an indication to perform a fetal magnetic resonance [3–6]. It allows to evaluate not only the presence or absence of liver in the thoracic cavity, but also to quantify the observed/expected total fetal lung volume (or/and TFLV), which was a better predictor in terms of postnatal survival. As an alternative to magnetic resonance evaluation of the or/and TFLV, some authors have demonstrated a close relationship between the liver herniation, the position of the stomach (which being anechoic is much more easily identifiable) and the postnatal outcome. Finally, given the high frequency with which EDC is associated with cardiovascular anomalies, there is an indication to perform fetal echocardiography [7, 8].

4.2 Antenatal therapies

The prenatal management of fetuses affected by CDH essentially provides for an ultrasound monitoring of the ultrasound parameters described above, associated in doubtful cases with second level examinations such as resonance. In recent years, however, fetal therapy has become increasingly popular on the international scene, indicated in cases where negative prognostic factors are detected in screening investigations (liver herniation, LHR <1.0). The purpose of these interventions is essentially to stop the mechanisms that induce the onset of complications such as pulmonary hypoplasia and pulmonary hypertension as early as possible. The technique currently most used is fetal tracheal occlusion (FETO): it is based on the principle that the occlusion of the trachea prevents the leakage of fluids, increasing the pressure in the airways and promoting lung growth. However, animal models have shown that tracheal occlusion reduces the maturation of type II pneumocytes, inducing a surfactant deficiency: for this reason the so-called “plug-unplug” sequence was devised, in which the patency of the trachea is first interrupted by the introduction of a balloon (or plug) and then re-established before delivery to allow lung maturation. This procedure can be performed percutaneously under ultrasound guidance or fetoscopy, typically between 27 and 32 weeks of gestational age, with the plug removed at 34 weeks. This procedure appears to be associated with increased survival in children with moderate and severe CDH, although further risk-benefit studies are certainly needed.

In children with CDH, the only medical treatment for which there is evidence of efficacy is corticosteroid therapy: maternal administration of one or two doses of corticosteroids at 34–36 weeks of gestation appears to be correlated with a reduction in respiratory morbidity at birth. Promising studies are also underway on the prenatal use of retinoids and phosphodiesterase inhibitors (Sildenafil) and on the use of stem cells from amniotic fluid in combination with FETO [4].

5. Postnatal management

The optimal timing and modality of delivery for children with CDH are still under discussion today. There seem to be no indications for induced delivery before 38 weeks of gestation, as well as there do not seem to be any advantages in performing a cesarean section. On the other hand, a unanimous consensus was found on the importance of planning the birth in a third-level center, where a multidisciplinary group (gynecologists, neonatologists, surgeons and pediatric anesthetists) is available, capable of managing the disease [4].

At birth, the main objective must be to ensure adequate ventilatory support (without triggering a vasospasm or further lung damage) and induce not too deep sedation (which would further compromise respiratory function). In case of respiratory distress, endotracheal intubation is carried out directly: in fact, ventilation with a facial mask must be avoided, as it would lead to distension of the stomach and intestinal loops, worsening the respiratory dynamics.

For the same principle, the positioning of a nasogastric tube is indicated at the same time, in order to decompress the stomach as much as possible. It is considered acceptable to maintain reduced saturation levels and a certain degree of hypercapnia, as long as the pH is kept above 7.2: in the presence of acidosis, in fact, vascular resistance would increase and consequently the risk of pulmonary hypertension. Another major problem in these patients is hemodynamic instability: to assess the need for inotropic support, these patients must be continuously monitored from a pressure point of view and postnatal echocardiography (within 48 h of life) must be performed if necessary repeated at 2–3 weeks. The indication for the ECMO, as a bridge to surgery in the most compromised patients, is still much debated. One of the biggest challenges remains the management of pulmonary hypertension: currently the most widely used treatment is inhaled nitric oxide, although encouraging new studies are underway on the use of Sildenafil [2, 4, 5].

Surgical treatment of CDH should be planned in election, after the achievement of hemodynamic stability. The only case in which it is acceptable to perform an emergency operation is when there are signs of ischemia of the herniated intestinal loops. As for the surgical technique, this can be performed openly (in thoracotomy or laparotomy) or by minimally invasive techniques. The intervention consists in the repositioning of the herniated organs within the abdomen and consequently in the closure of the defect, which can be primary or with a patch depending on the size of the defect. Minimally invasive techniques and the use of a patch were associated with a higher relapse rate [3, 4].

6. Long-term outcomes

In light of the increased survival of newborns with CDH, long-term outcomes, especially in terms of quality of life, have assumed increasing importance over time. The most compromised organs are certainly the lungs: in addition to the well-known pulmonary hypertension, these children experience alterations both in a restrictive sense (due to pulmonary hypoplasia) and in an obstructive sense (similar to bronchodysplasia of the premature infant) [8]. Pulmonary function seems to gradually restore during childhood, but recent studies have shown a slight deterioration of the same from childhood to adulthood. The respiratory system is not the only one affected by this disease. Gastroesophageal reflux is present in 45–89% of children with CDH and appears to be correlated with the size of the defect. Stunted growth is also a frequent finding, affecting 69% of these children at 1 year of age. Neurological alterations (in terms of delay in neurodevelopment but also sensorineural deafness) represent one of the most feared and also most frequent complications of CDH, with incidence rates ranging from 12 to 77%, especially in children undergoing ECMO. Finally, musculoskeletal deformities (chest anomalies, hemithorax asymmetries, scoliosis) were reported in 21–48% of patients treated for CDH [3].

All this, together with the fact that a good percentage of CDHs fall into syndromic pictures or are associated with other congenital anomalies, justifies the importance of a long-term follow-up program.

Author details

Marina Sica*, Carlotta Plessi and Francesco Molinaro
University of Siena, Italy

*Address all correspondence to: sicamarina121@gmail.com

References

[1] Lima M, editor. Pediatric Thoracic Surgery [Internet]. Mailand: Springer-Verlag; 2013 [cited 2021 Mar 27]. Available from: https://www.springer.com/gp/book/9788847052017

[2] Dingeldein M. Congenital diaphragmatic hernia. Advances in Pediatrics. 2018;**65**(1):241-247

[3] Leeuwen L, Fitzgerald DA. Congenital diaphragmatic hernia: Congenital diaphragmatic hernia. Journal of Paediatrics and Child Health. 2014;**50**(9):667-673

[4] Bloss RS, Aranda JV, Beardmore HE. Congenital diaphragmatic hernia: Pathophysiology and pharmacologic support. Surgery. 1981;**89**(4):518-524

[5] Kirby E, Keijzer R. Congenital diaphragmatic hernia: Current management strategies from antenatal diagnosis to long-term follow-up. Pediatric Surgery International. 2020;**36**(4):415-429

[6] Cordier A-G, Russo FM, Deprest J, Benachi A. Prenatal diagnosis, imaging, and prognosis in congenital diaphragmatic hernia. Seminars in Perinatology. 2020;**44**(1):51163

[7] Kitano Y. Prenatal intervention for congenital diaphragmatic hernia. Seminars in Pediatric Surgery. 2007;**16**(2):101-108

[8] Nakajima Y, Einspieler C, Marschik PB, Bos AF, Prechtl HFR. Does a detailed assessment of poor repertoire general movements help to identify those infants who will develop normally? Early Human Development. 2006;**82**(1):53-59

Chapter 7

Fetal Craniospinal Malformations: Aetiology and Diagnosis

Artur Beke, Virág Bartek and Aténé Simonyi

Abstract

The chapter discusses the aetiology and diagnostics of each fetal craniospinal disorder, particularly neural tube defects, ventriculomegaly, Dandy-Walker and Arnold-Chiari malformation, corpus callosum dysgenesis, iniencephaly, holoprosencephaly, microcephaly and kinked-brainstem. We aimed to highlight the usual ultrasound findings and genetic testing options.

Keywords: neural tube defects, anencephaly, exencephaly, spina bifida, ventriculomegaly, encephalocele, hydrocephalus, Dandy-Walker, Arnold-Chiari, corpus callosum, iniencephaly, kinked-brainstem, holoprosencephaly, microcephaly

1. Introduction

Our knowledge of the genetic background of the development of neurodevelopmental disorders is evolving. Today, ultrasound is a gold-standard diagnostic method for diagnosing developmental disorders. In addition to teratogenic causes, an increasing genetic background is being recognised for more and more fetal disorders. In addition to ultrasound diagnostics, the aim of this chapter is to investigate the genetic diagnostics of developmental disorders affecting the nervous system. In the case of malformations involving multiple organ systems, we investigate what chromosomal abnormalities or gene mutations may underlie each multiple disorder.

2. Fetal craniospinal malformations

2.1 Neural tube defects. Anencephaly/exencephaly. Spina bifida. Encephalocele

2.1.1 Epidemiology

Neural tube defects are the second most common structural-developmental malformations [1]. If the failure of neural tube closure is at the cranial end of the developing embryo, the disorder occurs in the form of anencephaly (initially exencephaly), if the failure is more caudal than cranial, it occurs in the form of spina bifida.

The prevalence of neural tube defects (NTDs) is 0.5–2/1000 live births, showing a heterogeneous geographical and ethnic distribution [2]. A genetic cause can be identified in 20% of cases [3].

2.1.2 Fetal morphology and prognosis

The brain of an anencephalic fetus is missing or missing in large parts. The form localising only to the cranium is called meroacrania, and extending to the foramen magnum is called holoacrania. If the spinal cord is also affected, the disorder is called craniorachischis.

The most severe neural tube closure disorder is caused by abnormal closure of the cranial section of the neural tube [4]. Anencephaly is a condition incompatible with life.

Spina bifida develops due to an abnormality in the closure of the neural tube caudally from the cranium. It basically affects the spinal region, with or without nerve tissue involvement. Its mildest form is spina bifida occulta, which is a defect of the vertebral arcs without affecting the underlying nerve tissue, most commonly in the sacral region, and usually causes no symptoms. In the case of spina bifida cystica, the lesion advances cystically. It can be closed (covered with skin or an opaque membrane) or open. If the cyst has meninx and cerebrospinal fluid but no nerve tissue in it, the lesion is called meningocele, if it also contains nerve tissue elements, the term is myelomeningocele [5]. The most severe form is myeloschisis (also known as rachischisis), which is an open lesion, so nothing covers the medullary (neural) plate [5]. After birth, spina bifida occulta usually does not cause symptoms, while spina bifida cystica can lead to paralysis of the lower extremities and urinary problems. Although myelomeningocele is a developmental disorder compatible with life, it is often associated with varying degrees of disability.

In encephalocele, the brain tissue with or without the meninges protrudes hernia-like through a pathological opening in the skull [5]. The most common site of its formation is os occipital [6]. Based on the grouping of Suwanwela and Suwanwela: cranial, frontoethmoidal, and basal encephalocele can be distinguished in addition to the occipital group [7].

2.1.3 Aetiology

To date, no clear genetic defect has been identified in the background of the development of NTDs, however, the role of a number of environmental and genetic predisposing factors is already known. It has been clinically demonstrated that folic acid supplementation significantly reduces the incidence of neural tube defects during the first trimester of pregnancy. Folic acid enrichment of the flour reduced the incidence of NTDs by 18% in 59 countries [8]. Folic acid, which is involved in purine and pyrimidine synthesis, is one of the cornerstones of DNA synthesis. Of course, not only isolated folic acid deficiency but any drug involved in folic acid synthesis may be associated with the development of anencephaly and other neural tube defects. These drugs such as antiepileptics (valproate or carbamazepine) and antimalarials (trimethoprim) are contraindicated during pregnancy without adequate folic acid supplementation, especially, in the first trimester.

In 1999, Shields et al. identified a heat-labile *MTHFR* C677T mutant gene that was present in the homozygous form of TT in 51 (18.8%) of 271 infants with neural tube defects (the homozygous form of CC did not increase the rate, whereas the heterozygous form of CT alone non-significantly increased the incidence of neural tube defects) [9].

Two members of the *SHROOM* gene family, the *SHROOM-2* and *SHROOM-3* genes have also been associated with the development of NTDs.

The role of the *SHROOM-3* gene in complex morphogenesis has long been demonstrated, and a mutation in a Loss of Function (LoF) (p.N594f) may be associated with the development of neural tube defects. The Shroom-3 protein encoded by the gene is involved in the planar cell polarity (PCP) pathway, and in animal models, it has been found that its main function is to regulate the distribution of myosin II in cells [10].

A Chinese research team, Z. Chen et al. isolated 1.56 times as many rare variants in the *SHROOM-3* gene in live-born children with NTD than in the control group. In addition, the same research has also linked another member of the *SHROOM* family, the *SHROOM-2* gene mutation, to the development of neural tube defects. *SHROOM-2* is a gene localised on the short arm of the X chromosome (Xp22.2), which encodes a protein of the same name, Shroom-2. Shroom-2 is expressed by endothelial cells; its role in facilitating the development of the contractile network in endothelial cells. In infants with NTD cases, 4.5 times as many deleterious missense (D-Mis) variants were identified compared with the control group. In the same study, *SHROOM-2* variants were found in 42 of the 343 NTD cases, of which 15 mutations were identified. More than one *SHROOM-2* mutation was found in five of these samples [1].

Because the convergent extension is a critical point in neural tube closure, mutation of the gene encoding any other protein in the PCP system that regulates it leads to neural tube closure disorders. Mutation of PCP core genes such as *VANGL2* or *CELSR1* has been shown in mouse models to lead to the development of severe NTDs [11]. It is likely that genes encoding other proteins involved in the PCP signalling pathway may also be associated with neural tube closure disorders, however, human orthologs of the genes found in the experimental models have not yet been identified, so this may be part of further research.

Foetuses of untreated diabetic mothers are also more prone to neural tube defects, as elevated blood glucose levels lead to misfolded proteins, their accumulation and apoptosis of cells through non-enzymatic glycosylation.

This causes structural damage to organogenesis, especially the neuroepithelium. In animal models, high-dose folic acid supplementation has also been shown to reduce the incidence of neural tube defects associated with high blood glucose [12]. In terms of other environmental factors, hyperthermia and vitamin A deficiency may also lead to NTD, the former due to heat stress and the latter due to its role in the retinoic acid pathway resulting in the inadequate closure of the neural tube. Maternal obesity increases the chances of developing NTDs through hyperinsulinemia, and metabolic syndrome through its teratogenic effect due to oxidative stress [13].

2.1.4 Diagnostics

Anencephaly can be diagnosed in the first trimester (in this case, exencephaly is shown in the image), but can only be diagnosed with ultrasound in the second trimester with high certainty, median time to prenatal diagnosis is 20 weeks (16–24) [14]. Ultrasound signals that the upper part of the skull is missing and that no parenchymal tissue can be detected in the skull, however, the brainstem and occipital bone can be identified. In the coronal plane, a 'frog eye' or 'Mickey Mouse' symptom is seen, which is due to a lack of cranial bones and a protruding bulbus. In some cases, it is associated with polyhydramnios, which is the result of insufficient amniotic fluid ingestion by the fetus.

Spina bifida can be diagnosed in the second trimester, with a median time of 21 weeks (18–24). The time and accuracy of detection depend largely on the type of spina bifida and the position of the fetus, as certain positions make it very difficult to follow the spinal column. The direct signs are the openness of the vertebral arches and herniation of the spinal cord, and the indirect signs are the lemon sign, the biconcave os frontale, and the banana sign, which is an abnormally bent, thin shape of the cerebellum. Ventriculomegaly due to cerebrospinal fluid flow disturbance is also common in foetuses with spina bifida, however, this ultrasound signal is not specific for diagnosis. Furthermore, the clivus-supraocciput angle is of diagnostic value; if it is less than 5 percentile, it raises the possibility of a form of neural tube defect associated with Chiari II malformation [15].

Thanks to modern technology, the availability of 3D and 4D ultrasound and MRI make it easier to diagnose neural tube defects so that in case of doubtful ultrasound findings, the diagnosis can be clarified by choosing another imaging modality. However, it should be noted that although these tests are much more accurate than conventional transabdominal and transvaginal ultrasound, their cost and limited availability make it essential to perform 2D ultrasound accurately and precisely, as it is still the most accessible, quickest and most economical method of diagnosis today.

In addition to imaging, laboratory tests can also support the diagnosis, as in 90% of cases, α-fetoprotein (AFP) levels are elevated in maternal blood and amniotic fluid, so this may be an additional tool to imaging. However, with the development of ultrasound, this test has been superseded.

In about one-tenth of cases, a chromosomal aberration or mutation has been identified as the cause of the neural tube defect, i.e., the majority of NTDs have a non-syndromic cause [16]. It can be seen that, although no clear environmental influence or genetic mutation has been identified as the cause of NTDs, it is likely that their development is multifactorial, i.e., genetic predisposing factors and environmental stresses contribute to their development.

2.1.5 Postnatal morphology and associated disorders

Postnatally, the anencephalic infant lacks a cranial bone (skull), the cerebellum is only a mass, shrunken. The ears are low set and deformed. Facial structures such as the eyes, nose and cheeks are large. The neck is short and spinal abnormalities may be present. The limbs are deformed, the thymus is abnormally large and pulmonary hypoplasia is often present. Spina bifida may be present with minimal external signs depending on the severity of the disease (in spina bifida occulta, only a darker patch or patch of hair-covered skin in the sacral region indicates a malformation). Depending on the region affected, a child with spina bifida lacks the structures covering the spinal column at the affected vertebrae and may have a herniated spinal cord; in meningocele and myelomeningocele, the protruding cyst is visible in the occipital region, with or without nerve tissue.

Neural tube defects are most commonly associated with renal abnormalities such as hydronephrosis, polycystic kidney disease, uni- or bilateral agenesis or unilateral hypoplasia. Cardiac malformations range from simple septal defects to complex cardiac malformations [17].

2.2 Congenital ventriculomegaly and hydrocephalus

2.2.1 Epidemiology

Ventriculomegaly is one of the most common pathological findings during antenatal ultrasound screening [18]. In severe cases, we are talking about hydrocephalus. The prevalence of hydrocephalus is 11/1000 live births [19].

2.2.2 Fetal morphology and prognosis

Hydrocephalus develops due to a progressive increase or impaired absorption of intraventricular cerebrospinal fluid (CSF) and its pathomechanism can be either obstructive or communicating [17, 20]. Increased pressure leads to the dilation of the ventricles, i.e., ventriculomegaly. If the brain volume thins due to the growth of the ventricles, we speak of hydrocephalus internus, if the volume of cerebrospinal fluid increases in the subarachnoid spaces, we speak of hydrocephalus externus. Macrocephaly can also develop with the growth of the bony skull [5], and the skull of such a fetus is larger than average.

The CSF is produced by the choroid plexus, circulates in the ventricles, then exits through the fourth ventricle into the subarachnoid space, where it is absorbed by the granulationes arachnoideae and finally drained through the venous sinuses into the systemic circulation. 1/3 of the CSF enters the lymphatic circulation, however, pathological alterations of this have not yet been demonstrated in human models [19].

The prognosis of hydrocephalus depends on its severity and the success of prenatal treatment. Of the 90 cases of hydrocephalus followed up by Yamasaki et al., 17% resulted in death, 21% were diagnosed with severe retardation, 13% with moderate retardation and 26% with mild retardation. A normal phenotype was described in 23% of cases [21].

The classification of ventriculomegaly depends on the degree of dilatation detected on ultrasound: mild ventriculomegaly between 10–12 mm, moderate ventriculomegaly between 13–15 mm and severe ventriculomegaly above 15 mm. The measurement is taken at the atrium of the lateral ventricle, the point where the temporal and posterior horns converge. This is a fixed value between 15 and 40 weeks of pregnancy [22].

If no abnormality is found in genetic testing and no other associated abnormality is present, mild ventriculomegaly is not considered pathological, and postnatally 90% of these cases present a normal phenotype, i.e., the wider ventricle is considered a normal variant [22].

2.2.3 Aetiology

Congenital hydrocephalus can be syndromic or non-syndromic, but in half of the cases, it is idiopathic [20]. The most common form of congenital hydrocephalus is the X-linked monogenic *L1CAM* mutation. The gene product of *L1CAM* is a protein that plays a key role in neuronal migration.

Hydrocephalus due to the *L1CAM* mutation is one of the most severe forms associated with stenosis of the aqueduct of Sylvius, known as HSAS (Hydrocephalus with Stenosis of the Aqueduct of Sylvius). It is often associated with corpus callosum agenesia or hypoplasia, adducted thumb and other structural cerebellar abnormalities [20]. Another form of X-linked congenital hydrocephalus is associated with *AP1S2* mutation [23].

Mutations in the *MPDZ* gene lead to primary ependymal malformations, including hydrocephalus [20]. *MPDZ* encodes a protein that regulates tight junction function and is also likely involved in the PCP pathway [24]. Mutations in this gene at 9p23 lead to autosomal recessive non-syndromic hydrocephalus [25]. Another form of autosomal recessive hydrocephalus is caused by mutations in *CCDC88C*. This gene encodes a protein called Daple, which interacts with Dishevelled protein to regulate cell migration. The Dishevelled protein is a member of the non-canonical Wnt pathway [26].

In addition to these well-studied genes, two others have recently been identified that are associated with the development of hydrocephalus. The *EML1* gene (14q32.2) encodes a microtubule system-related protein that is also involved in the PCP pathway. The gene mutation results in abnormal development of the posterior part of the skull, leading to severe hydrocephalus [23]. Also in this study, Shaheen et al. described another mutation, *WDR81* (17p13.3), which leads to severe hydrocephalus with cerebellar hypoplasia.

Neural tube defects are often associated with hydrocephalus. This may be due to common genetic factors and environmental aetiology, and pathological spinal development may itself be a physical barrier to CSF. Arachnoid cysts may also form a physical barrier in the pathway of cerebrospinal fluid. As arachnoid cysts occur in 15% of Phelan-McDermid syndromes, this syndrome is also often associated with hydrocephalus [19]. Other syndromes include mucopolysaccharidosis, Sotos syndrome and Rothmund-Thomson syndrome. Cytogenetic abnormalities have also been associated with the disorder, such as microdeletion of 9q22.3, partial trisomy of chromosome 1, but hydrocephalus is also common in Patau, Edwards and Down syndromes [19].

Ventriculomegaly/hydrocephalus may occur in isolated cases as a consequence of TORCH (Toxoplasma, Rubeola, Cytomegalovirus, Herpes simplex and other viruses) infection during pregnancy, or in rare cases due to congenital tumours such as choroid plexus papilloma [21].

2.2.4 Diagnostics

In terms of ultrasound diagnostics, it should be noted that in the first trimester, physiological ventricular dilatation is present, so hydrocephalus can only be diagnosed with certainty after the 14th week. The first characteristic ultrasound sign is asymmetry of the choroid plexus [27]. The top of the fourth ventricle may show an abnormal image and the absence of foramina Magendii and Luschka is common [17]. Due to the progressive nature of hydrocephalus, it may develop throughout pregnancy and even after birth without any previous ultrasound signal. Thus, the time to diagnosis also varies widely; Yamasaki et al., in their study of 156 cases of hydrocephalus, found the diagnosis to be made between 13 and 40 weeks (51% of cases were already diagnosed before 28 weeks). Breeze et al., also reported similar data, with a median time to diagnosis of 28 weeks (16–36) [28].

In addition to ultrasound, if ventriculomegaly or hydrocephalus is suspected, a Magnetic Resonance Imaging (MRI) scan may be useful, as it is a more accurate and reliable way of showing the development of brain structures and their possible malformations than ultrasound. However, it should be taken into account that, in addition to the general disadvantages of MRI (difficult availability, high costs), the fact that the fetal movement makes the findings more difficult or impossible to evaluate in antenatal diagnosis is a particular difficulty [29].

2.2.5 Postnatal morphology and associated disorders

The neonate with ventriculomegaly/hydrocephalus has macrocephaly, which may progress postnatally [30]. The disorder is often associated with neural tube defects due to common genetic predisposing factors.

2.3 Dandy-Walker malformation

2.3.1 Epidemiology

The incidence of this malformation is 0.33/1000 live births [31], i.e., it is a relatively rare disorder.

2.3.2 Fetal morphology and prognosis

The Dandy-Walker malformation includes dilatation of the fourth ventricle with hypoplasia or agenesis of the vermis of the cerebellum. A pseudocyst often develops at the base of the posterior fossa. Survival is low (about half of cases) [5].

2.3.3 Aetiology

Genetically heterogeneous in origin, several mutations have been described in recent years. However, one of the main "suspects" are the *ZIC1* and *ZIC4* genes, located at 3q24. In terms of inheritance, autosomal dominant, recessive and X-linked inheritance patterns have been reported, so it may be present as part of trisomy 9 (AR) or 6p (AD), but it may also be associated with Aicardi syndrome.

It is common in Edwards syndrome. However, in addition to genetic causes, a number of environmental factors may contribute to its development, such as maternal alcoholism or severe diabetes mellitus, as well as TORCH infection in the first trimester [17].

2.3.4 Diagnostics

Dandy-Walker malformation can be diagnosed by ultrasound at the earliest at week 11, but it should be noted that isolated dilatation of the fourth ventricle may be physiological during early development. In addition, the cerebellar vermis is not fully developed until the second trimester. In conclusion, an accurate diagnosis is only possible during the second trimester [27].

2.3.5 Postnatal morphology and associated disorders

Since the disorder mainly affects the cerebellum, in case of survival, postnatally the disorder may be marked by muscle movement disorders, learning difficulties and mental retardation. Hydrocephalus and consequent macrocephaly often develop due to inhibition of cerebrospinal fluid drainage [17]. It is often associated with hyperdactyly, syndactyly, renal, hepatic and pancreatic alloplasia and abnormal retina [32].

2.4 Arnold-Chiari malformation

2.4.1 Epidemiology

There are four types of Arnold-Chiari syndrome. Its prevalence is 0.9/1000 live births [33].

2.4.2 Fetal morphology and prognosis

In type I, the cerebellar tonsils are ectopic, with a part of the tonsils pressing into the foramen magnum, often in isolation. In type II, there is cerebellar hypoplasia with myelomeningocele, part of the tonsils and the elongated distal part of the brainstem protruding into the foramen magnum. In type III, the cerebellum is herniated due to the absence of occipital bone and spina bifida. In type IV, the most severe type, the cerebellum itself is hypoplastic [17]. Structural deformities lead to hydrocephalus. A lesion with a poor prognosis.

2.4.3 Aetiology

In the majority of cases, Arnold-Chiari malformation is multifactorial, and external environmental factors may also play a role in the development of the disease.

A precise genetic mutation has not yet been identified. It is assumed to be the result of mutations in proteins involved in the Sonic hedgehog and Wnt pathways, suggesting that there is an overlap at the gene level between mutations causing neural tube defects and Arnold-Chiari malformation, but this requires further research. Its aetiology is probably multifactorial and it cannot be ruled out that various environmental factors also contribute to the development of the phenotype.

Syringomyelia is often described in this pathology. In syringomyelia, the cavity formation observed in the nervous system may be due to residual formations from embryonic age, but may also occur as a result of haemorrhage or inflammation.

2.4.4 Diagnostics

An ultrasound scan in the second trimester of pregnancy can raise suspicion of the lesion, and if necessary, an MRI scan can confirm the diagnosis.

2.4.5 Postnatal morphology and associated disorders

Type I occurs in 3–5% of patients with Klippel-Feil syndrome, suggesting that abnormal *GDF6* and *GDF3* function may also be associated with the development of the syndrome [33].

Syringomyelia, which is often associated with type II, is rarely hereditary and may be associated with the following additional pathological conditions and gene mutations: hydrocephalus (*NF1, NES, GFAP, FGFR2, AQP4*), spina bifida (*GDF6, GDF3*) and other spinal deformities (*VDR, POC5, NF1, GH1, GFAP, GDF3*), various neurological tumours: astrocytoma (*NRAS, NF1, NES, GFAP, COL1A1*), neurilemmoma (*NF1, NES, GFAP*), ependymoma (*NES, GFAP*).

In addition, syringomyelia may also be caused by tissue weakness, such as in Ehlers-Danlos syndrome (mutations in *COL1A1, COL1A2, COL3A1, COL5A1, COL5A2, TNXB, ADAMTS2, PLOD1, B4GALT7, DSE, D4ST1/CHST14* genes) or Marfan syndrome (mutation in *FBN1* gene).

2.5 Corpus callosum agenesia/dysgenesis

2.5.1 Epidemiology

The prevalence of malformations of the corpus callosum is 0.25/1000 live births. In terms of aetiology, 30–45% of cases are due to genetic causes, 10% to chromosomal abnormalities and 20–35% are associated with a genetic syndrome. In some cases, environmental factors (e.g., maternal alcohol consumption) also lead to corpus callosum dys- or agenesis [34].

2.5.2 Fetal morphology and prognosis

The corpus callosum is one of the five major cerebral commissures and is one of the largest white matter-containing tract in the brain. Its role is to connect the right and left hemispheres of the brain, and it is thought that 2–3% of the cortical fibres are passing through it. Its main function is to coordinate the hemispheres of the brain and to integrate sensory and motor functions [35].

Isolated corpus callosum dys- or agenesis is a disorder compatible with life, however, approximately 25% of foetuses with isolated corpus callosum agenesis/dysgenesis diagnosed antenatally will later have an intellectual disability. In addition, mild social or learning deficits may occur even with normal intelligence [35]. If the developmental disorder is part of a syndrome, the outcome of the disease depends on the particular syndrome.

2.5.3 Aetiology

Known chromosomal abnormalities affect chromosomes 1, 4, 6, 8 and 17. The most common type is a deletion, including the 1q42-q44 deletion causing corpus callosum dys- or agenesis of variable severity [35]. As most of the proteins encoded by these regions regulate or are involved in a key moment in nervous system development, corpus callosum dys- or agenesis as an isolated developmental disorder does not occur in any of the chromosomal disorders, but is often associated with microcephaly, hydrocephalus or craniofacial abnormalities.

Inheritance patterns include autosomal dominant, recessive and X-linked hereditary syndromes.

A very severe form of X-linked dominant (XLD) inheritance is Aicardi syndrome, which is incompatible with life in male foetuses but also has high premature mortality in girls. In addition to corpus callosum agenesis, it is associated with infantile seizures (infantile spasm) and the development of chorioretinal lacunes [36].

The autosomal dominant form is frontonasal dysplasia, Goldenhar syndrome; autosomal recessive form is Andermann syndrome, craniotelencephalic dysplasia, Da Silva or Leigh syndrome. Isolated corpus callosum dys- or agenesis can be inherited in an autosomal recessive, X-linked recessive (XLR) or autosomal recessive (AR) manner [17].

2.5.4 Diagnostics

Developmental abnormalities of the corpus callosum are difficult to detect before 18 weeks [35]. Ultrasonography shows colpocephaly, a high-lying enlarged third ventricle with absent or abnormal morphology of the corpus callosum [34]. These may confirm the suspicion, as in ultrasound diagnostics there is always the question of whether the absence of a formula is not only due to the position of the fetus, or possibly to a technician error. In their 2012 study, Santo et al. found that the number of false-positive ultrasound findings can be as high as 20%. An MRI scan after 22 weeks can confirm or refute the ultrasound findings with high certainty [37].

2.5.5 Post-natal morphology and associated abnormalities

Corpus callosum dys- or agenesis is often associated with microcephaly, hydrocephalus or craniofacial abnormalities [17]. Therefore, both the postnatal picture and the associated abnormalities are influenced by the gene mutation that results in the disorder.

2.6 Holoprosencephaly

2.6.1 Epidemiology

Holoprosencephaly is a midline malformation of the cranium and face. Its prevalence is estimated to be between 0.2 and 0.06 per 1000 live births [17, 38].

2.6.2 Fetal morphology and prognosis

The three main types of holoprosencephaly are lobar, semi-lobar and alobar. The most severe form is alobar, where midline separation is completely absent and the blister of the telencephalon does not separate. Typically, the corpus callosum and the third ventricle are absent, and cyclopia and proboscis are present. In the semilobar form, the frontal and parietal lobes are usually not separated bilaterally, but all septations, especially in the posterior region, are observed. Microphtalmia or anophtalmia, nasal malformations may also be associated. In the least severe form, the lobar form, the two hemispheres are essentially retained, with varying degrees of fusion between the two halves. The nose may be depressed with eyes sitting close, but the facial phenotype may be completely normal [39].

The prognosis depends on the severity of the holoprosencephaly. Mortality is high in alobar cases.

2.6.3 Aetiology

As with all neural tube defects, the development of holoprosencephaly is multifactorial, with both genetic and environmental influences contributing to its occurrence [40].

It is often associated with chromosomal abnormalities, most commonly with trisomy (Patau syndrome) or deletion of chromosome 13, but may also be associated with trisomy and deletion of chromosomes 18 and 21. Monogenic syndromes have also been associated with foetuses with holoprosencephaly, such as ARH (autosomal recessive holoprosencephaly), ADH (autosomal dominant holoprosencephaly), Váradi-Papp syndrome (AR), Grote syndrome (AR), Steinfield syndrome (AD) or holoprosencephaly-fetal akinesia syndrome (XL) (Wainwright, 2005). Environmental influences have also been implicated in the development of holoprosencephaly, such as maternal alcohol consumption during pregnancy and insulin-dependent diabetes mellitus.

A clear genetic mutation has been identified in the background of 15–20% of holoprosencephalic disorders [41]. Since the Sonic hedgehog signalling pathway is responsible for the regulation of the ventral phase of nervous system development and for the separation of the brain vesicles, it is understandable that genes affecting this mutation and their dysfunctional protein products would also be involved in this pathway. Mutations in the *SHH* gene itself have been demonstrated to underlie holoprosencephalic retardation since 1996 [42]. Later, mutations in several members of the signalling pathway were identified, including mutations in *PTCH1* and *GLI2*. The Six-3 protein has not yet been linked to any of the signalling pathways, but mutations in *SIX3* are responsible for about 1.3% of holoprosencephaly cases. Six-3 is thought to play a role in the Wnt pathway [43].

There are also correlations between the development of neural tube defects and holoprosencephaly due to their common predisposing factors. K. Shiota found 14 cases of exencephaly or myeloschisis in 150 embryos with holoprosencephaly, but no correlation was found between holoprosencephaly and the severity of the neural tube defect. Diabetic mothers have a higher risk of developing both holoprosencephaly and neural tube defects [41].

2.6.4 Diagnostics

It can be diagnosed prenatally by transabdominal or transvaginal ultrasound, however, some of the milder lobar forms are difficult to diagnose by ultrasound. The median time to diagnosis of holoprosencephaly is 12 weeks (10–14) [27]. In the alobar type, morphological abnormalities of the face (cyclopia, ethmocephaly, cebocephaly) and absence of the choroid plexus in the lateral ventricles are well diagnosed by ultrasound. Dorsal cysts, ventriculomegaly and absence of the cavum septum pellucidum may also be associated findings [44]. An ultrasound sign of semilobar holoprosencephaly is incomplete separation of the hemispheric nuclei and fused thalamus. Both types are often associated with polydactyly, renal dysplasia, omphalocele and hydrops [44].

2.6.5 Postnatal morphology and associated disorders

Kaliaperumal et al. found a 95% mortality rate in alobar holoprosencephaly after antenatal diagnosis. Even mild cases are associated with severe postnatal complications, often requiring neurosurgery and intensive care [45].

2.7 Microcephaly

2.7.1 Epidemiology

Microcephaly is a deviation of at least three standard deviations of head circumference from the mean for given sex and age at fetal maturity [46]. A microcephaly finding is a clinical finding in itself, not a diagnosis [47]. Primary microcephaly is defined as a diagnosis made before 36 weeks of gestation, secondary microcephaly develops after birth [47]. The incidence of primary microcephaly is 0.16–0.025/1000 live births [17].

2.7.2 Fetal morphology and prognosis

Primary microcephaly is a static condition [48]. Phenotypic microcephaly is associated with varying degrees of cognitive deficits depending on the mutation, in addition, to head circumferential abnormalities, but weight, height and other external variations are not common. Imaging studies show normal brain morphology [48]. The prognosis depends on the type of mutation and is generally good, but in the majority of cases, severe deterioration in the quality of life is to be expected.

2.7.3 Aetiology

In terms of aetiology, microcephaly may be caused by a reduction or absence of neurogenesis (due to Cytomegalovirus (CMV) infection, chromosomal abnormality or primary autosomal recessive microcephaly), a prenatal destructive process (e.g., hypoxia, ischaemia) or a rare genetic syndrome.

TORCH infection suffered antenatally, especially in the first trimester, also increases the chance of developing microcephaly [47]. In addition to TORCH pathogens, the Zika virus has received particularly high press coverage in recent years due to the increased number of cases in the US. The association between Zika virus infection during pregnancy and primary microcephaly was quickly shown to be significant. 41,473 pregnant women infected with Zika virus were studied in Brazil between 2015 and 2016. Of these, 1950 cases of microcephaly associated with infection were recorded [49]. The almost 5% case rate is a huge increase compared to the average of 0.02%, and therefore more attention should be paid to mapping the teratogenic effects of Zika virus and preventing infection.

In particular, exposure to harmful substances such as maternal alcohol consumption in the first trimester increases the risk of developing microcephaly in addition to neural tube defects and hydrocephalus. Since fetal hypoxia during pregnancy can also lead to the development of microcephaly, special attention should be paid to pregnant women with placental insufficiency [47].

Isolated microcephaly is an autosomal recessively inherited disorder. Its pathomechanism is a disorder of neurogenic tissue mitotic activity, with normal cell migration and apoptosis [48]. Currently, 18 genes have been identified in the pathogenesis of primary microcephaly. All are members of the MCPH (autosomal recessive primary microcephaly) gene family.

In addition to the autosomal recessive form, mutations in other gene families are known to lead to primary microcephaly. These include *KIF2A, KIF5C* and *KIF11* from the kinesin family, and *TUBG1, TUBB2B* and *TUBA1A* from the tubulin family. The proteins encoded by these genes also contribute to the physiological function of the microtubule system.

Among chromosomal abnormalities, microcephaly is often associated with Patau, Edwards and Down syndromes [17].

2.7.4 Diagnostics

Ultrasound diagnosis is made by calculating the head circumference, calculated from the biparietal diameter and the occipitofrontal diameter. This derived value is compared with the mean value for the developmental stage and sex, and if it is at least two [50], in other sources three [46], standard deviations lower than the mean, it raises the possibility of microcephaly.

However, it is worth noting that individual variations may occur without organic deviation, and therefore further examinations to exclude false positivity is always important in the diagnosis of microcephaly. Other imaging, MRI, 3D or 4D ultrasound may be helpful. If a genetic abnormality is suspected, depending on the gestational age, amniocentesis and detailed genetic testing should be considered, especially if microcephaly is associated with other suspected signs (e.g. Intrauterine Growth Restriction, IUGR).

2.7.5 Postnatal morphology and associated disorders

Microcephaly may be associated with certain syndromes. One of these is the autosomal recessive Meier-Gorlin syndrome, which is caused by mutations in the *ORC1, ORC4, and ORC6, CDT1* or *CDC6* gene. The syndrome is one of the primordial dwarfisms and is characterised by intrauterine growth retardation, absence of patella, small ears and microcephaly. Pulmonary emphysema is common [51]. Other notable conditions include Nijmegen-Breakage syndrome, Ligase IV syndrome, Warsaw-Breakage syndrome, severe combined immunodeficiency (SCID) or Bloom syndrome [52].

2.8 Sacrococcygeal teratoma

2.8.1 Epidemiology

Sacrococcygeal teratoma is the most common neonatal tumour with a prevalence of 0.027/1000 live births. Its origin is pluripotent cell proliferation with tissue from all three germinal discs. The origin of the cells is remnant cells of the primitive streak or primordial germ cells [53]. It is more common in female foetuses, with a 4:1 ratio [54].

2.8.2 Fetal morphology and prognosis

The typical site of the tumour is the sacral region, hence its name, and it can often grow very large. In terms of pathology, it can be benign (mature) or malignant (immature). The majority of tumours (90%) are benign [55]. The tumour may be cystic or solid, as well as mixed in appearance. Often it may degenerate secondarily, calcify, or may contain haemorrhagic or necrotic regions [55].

The Altman classification was established based on the anatomical location of the tumour. Altman I is largely located externally, II has an associated intrapelvic tumour, III is largely located in the abdominal cavity, and IV is predominantly located presacrally, often without an externally visible tumour [56].

At prenatal diagnosis, the prognosis is poor, with frequent intrauterine death, mainly due to cardiac failure. In contrast, the prognosis is excellent after surgical intervention for postnatally diagnosed sacrococcygeal teratomas [54].

2.8.3 Aetiology

Sacrococcygeal teratoma is rarely associated with chromosomal abnormalities. There is literature evidence that sacrococcygeal teratoma can be associated with partial 13q22 trisomy [57]. Mutations associated with the 12p region are common in adult germ cell tumours, but this mutation has not been detected in "pure" sacrococcygeal teratomas [58]. However, the 12p mutation is common in sacrococcygeal teratomas where a yolk sac component is also present in the tumour. Based on this, Emans et al. suggest that sacrococcygeal teratomas should be classified into two groups depending on the absence or presence of the 12p isochromosome [59].

Rarely, sacrococcygeal teratoma may be part of the Currarino triad. It is an autosomal dominant inherited disorder with mutations in the *HLXB9* gene in the 7q36 region and is associated with anorectal malformations and presacral tissue proliferation and tumours in addition to teratoma. Presacral tumours associated with the Currarino triad have a much lower chance of malignancy than non-syndromic forms [60].

In other rare cases, it may be associated with 3q trisomy, resulting in a Cornelia de Lange syndrome-like phenotype (short stature, bone developmental malformations, mental retardation, facial developmental abnormalities) [59].

2.8.4 Diagnostics

One of the most important suspicious signs is a larger uterus compared to the gestational age. This is caused by the size of the tumour or by the associated polyhydramnios. The visible tumour mass required to confirm the suspicion may be seen on ultrasound from as early as week 13, but its differential diagnosis is difficult, as the visible mass in the sacral region may also be pseudocyst, obstructive uropathy or meconium. In such cases, as is often the case in neurodevelopmental disorders, it is worthwhile to have an additional MRI scan.

An enlarged placenta and/or fetal hydrops may cause the mother to develop a condition similar to eclampsia, maternal mirror syndrome.

2.8.5 Postnatal morphology and associated disorders

The American Academy of Paediatrics Surgical Section (AAPSS) has developed a classification system that allows inferring the chance of malignancy and future complications depending on the presence of presacral and external tumours, the diagnosis, the success of the resection. In the I to IV scheme, grade I is the mildest with the least tendency to malignancy, while grade IV is the most severe and most likely to malign [55].

Associated abnormalities are usually consequential, so obstruction of the urinary tract, hydronephrosis, rectal atresia, bony malformation of the sacral region as well as fetal hydrops may occur [55]. Hip dysplasia and hydronephrosis may also be associated with sacrococcygeal teratoma in an unconsequential manner, so screening for these is essential both ante- and postnatally [56].

2.9 Kinked brainstem

2.9.1 Epidemiology

Kinked brainstem is an extremely rare condition. It is often only recognised postnatally. Precise figures on its incidence are not yet available.

2.9.2 Fetal morphology and prognosis

A kinked brainstem (twisted brainstem, fractured brainstem, also known as a Z-shaped brainstem) is a rare lesion, a sign of severe neurodysgenesis [61] on pre- or postnatal brain MRI scans. It usually occurs in association with other neurodevelopmental disorders and has a poor prognosis [62].

The posterior fossa is formed early during gestation. Brainstem folding occurs between the third and eighth week, with cerebellum development complete by the 16th week of gestation. Between the third and fifth week, the forebrain folds in accordance with the developing brainstem structures, creating the flexura cephalica, flexura pontis and flexura cervicalis. In the kinked brainstem, the angle of the flexures is increased, normal brainstem and cerebellar development are inhibited, and cerebellar hypoplasia is, therefore, an associated abnormality in almost all cases [61].

2.9.3 Aetiology

So far, three syndromes have been identified in which kinked brainstem is present as an associated disorder: alpha-dystroglycanopathies (e.g., Walker-Warburg syndrome), tubulinopathies and X-linked hydrocephalus.

Alpha-dystroglycanopathies are heterogeneous congenital muscular dystrophies with brain, muscle and eye involvement [63]. At the more severe end of the spectrum is autosomal recessive Walker-Warburg syndrome, a defect in O-mannosyltransferase. It is often associated with ocular abnormalities (e.g. microphthalmia, retinal detachment), but these can often only be diagnosed after birth. Other alpha-dystroglycanopathies include muscle-eye-brain disease, Fukuyama muscular and cerebral dystrophy and muscle-eye-brain disease with bilateral multicystic leukodystrophy.

Alpha-dystroglycanopathy may be suspected if cobblestone lissencephaly is present. The trunks may be enlarged. Encephalocele is not a diagnostic criterion but may confirm suspicion [61, 62].

The genes identified so far that cause alpha-dystroglycanopathy are *FKRP, FKTN, POMT1, POMT2, POMGnT1, LARGE, ISPD, GTDC2, DAG1, TMEM5, B3GALNT2, B3GNT1, GMPPB, SGK196, DPM1, DPM2, DPM3, DOLK* [64].

There are two types of tubolinopathy, a more severe and a milder form. The more severe form is associated with microlissencephaly and 'kinked brainstem', the milder form is associated with more non-specific nervous system abnormalities. Three genes have been identified so far in its background: *TUBA1A* (chromosome 12), *TUBB2B* (chromosome 6) and *TUBB3* (chromosome 16) [65].

X-linked hydrocephalus is caused by the *L1CAM* (X-chromosome) mutation. It is suspected if the fetus is a boy and the cerebral aqueduct is not detectable on MRI even with a high T2 signal (however, this is difficult to diagnose if the fetus is small or moves around a lot during the scan). Spasticity and adduction of the thumbs may be associated (mainly seen on dynamic ultrasound, but not a diagnostic criterion). Usually, the hemispheres and trunks are not affected by the lesion [62].

2.9.4 Diagnostics

The abnormality is usually diagnosed prenatally during an MRI scan for suspected ventriculomegaly or other intracranial lesions. If the anomaly has not been diagnosed prenatally, a newborn with a kinked brainstem will require intensive care and will be in poor condition. Regardless of the associated abnormalities, the newborn presents with a variety of neurological symptoms, hypotonia and seizures [62].

2.9.5 Postnatal morphology and associated disorders

The kinked brainstem refers to the increase in the angle of the pontomesencephalic transition, exact figures have not been described so far. The brainstem may dislocate posteriorly or anteriorly at the midbrain bridge level. It is often associated with other intracranial abnormalities. Cerebellar hypoplasia is almost always present.

Other associated abnormalities may include ventriculomegaly, dys- or agenesis of the corpus callosum, delayed cortical development, neuron migration disorders (e.g., lissencephaly), Dandy-Walker malformation, vertex encephalocele, abnormal cerebral hemispheres or abnormal head size (micro- or macrocephaly) [61].

Polymicrogyria and cobblestone lissencephaly are strongly suggestive of alpha-dystroglycanopathy, but the assessment of neuronal migration is difficult prenatally because the fetal brain is brainstem-rich until about 16 weeks gestation. Cerebellar cysts may also be present, however, these do not develop until the second week after birth [63].

The complicating factor is the secondary damage to cortical structures due to preexisting ventriculomegaly and hydrocephalus.

In a review of seven cases, Stroustrup et al. found that in two cases, the "kinked brainstem" was misidentified as a cerebellum on ultrasound [61]. Since the posterior fossa and the brainstem area are difficult to examine by ultrasound, it is advisable to request an MRI scan in case of a suspicious finding.

Theoretically, the abnormality can be diagnosed from week 7, but in practice, it is usually detected during the second-trimester screening.

2.10 Iniencephaly

2.10.1 Epidemiology

Iniencephaly is a complex malformation characterised by the absence of a neck, pronounced cervicothoracic lordosis and spina bifida.

Its prevalence is very rare and varies between 1 and 0.02/1000 live births, however, the actual prevalence may be higher, as iniencephaly is not always described as part of complex disorders [66].

2.10.2 Fetal morphology and prognosis

It is characterised by the complete or partial absence of the os occipital scales and of the cervical and thoracic vertebrae, an irregular fusion of the existing vertebrae and absence of the neck due to abnormalities in the closure of the vertebral arch. The foramen magnum is wider, while the posterior fossa is usually smaller. Due to the high degree of lordosis of the cervicothoracic spinal segment, the head is strongly tilted backwards, the face is upward (so-called "stargazing") and the trunk is shortened. It is often associated with other neural tube defects, open spina bifida or anencephaly. The disease has a very poor prognosis. If born alive, the newborn dies within a few hours (although one case has been described where the affected individual survived to adulthood and retained his or her intellect) [67].

We distinguish between two types of iniencephaly, iniencephaly apertus (with encephalocele) and iniencephaly clausus (without encephalocele) [68].

2.10.3 Aetiology

Its occurrence is predominantly sporadic. It is more common in female foetuses. Environmental effects have been described in association with maternal syphilis and drug intoxication. Chen et al. found chromosomal abnormalities in 5 of 16 cases studied (two cases of trisomy 18, two cases of trisomy of chromosome 13 mosaic and one case of monosomy of chromosome X mosaic) [66].

Since this is a type of neural tube defect, adequate folate supplementation can reduce the chances of its development, and all the factors described above as leading to the development of neural tube defects also contribute to the development of iniencephaly.

2.10.4 Diagnostics

Cuillier et al. diagnosed iniencephaly by transvaginal ultrasound at the 9th gestational week as the earliest on the basis of acrania, encephalocele and shortened spine [69]. Iniencephaly can be diagnosed with certainty from gestational week 13. Ultrasound signs include extreme dorsiflexion of the head, abnormally short and deformed spine and occipital meningocele. Polyhydramnios is always present.

In terms of differential diagnosis, it should be distinguished from cervical hyperextension, prenatal teratoma, lymphangioma, cervical myelomeningocele, Klipper-Feil and Jarcho-Levin syndromes.

Klipper-Feil syndrome is caused by a failure of segmentation of the cervical vertebrae early in gestation. There is no spina bifida in this case. There are usually associated neurological symptoms, often associated with deafness. Most cases are sporadic, but autosomal dominant and recessive forms have been described [66]. Klipper-Feil syndrome can be subsequently treated surgically [68].

2.10.5 Postnatal morphology and associated disorders

In 84% of cases, other anomalies are also associated: anencephaly, encephalocele, hydrocephalus, cyclopia, mandibular defect, cleft lip and palate, cardiovascular anomalies, diaphragmatic hernia, omphalocele, gastroschisis, situs inversus, ren polycysticum, arthrogriposis. It may also be associated with an undescribed frequency of Dandy-Walker malformation, hydronephrosis, atresia of the gastrointestinal system and umbilical artery singularis [66].

2.11 The epigenetics of fetal craniospinal malformations

As the cause of craniospinal malformations is usually multifactorial, it is understandable that epigenetic pathways should play an important role in neurulation, although it is yet a poorly researched area. The relation between neural tube defects and epigenetic pathways is the most studied part.

Multiple ways have been identified which affect the formation of neural tubes epigenetically. The most reviewed topic is DNA methylation, although only animal studies are available. In DNA methyltransferases *DNMT3A* and *DNMT3B* knocked-out mice neural tube defects are more common. It is also possible that *DNMT3L* plays a role in the process too, although it is less researched [70]. Mouse models have also been made to examine histone acetyltransferases, and it has been identified that histone acetyltransferases *GCN5* and *CBP* are both play a significant role in neurulation. It is supposed that it has an impact on human neural tube development too. Nucleosome positioning, another example of epigenetic regulation, is also studied in association with NTDs, as a subtype of ATP-dependent chromatin remodelling complex, the SWI/SNF-related nucleosome remodelling BAF complex has been proved to play an important role in the relation of neural tube closing in mice. Also, micro RNAs, like CECR2 have been proven to cause exencephaly in animal models [71].

It is clear that the epigenetic pathways do not function on their own, but rather as a part of a complex system. It would be important to examine and understand more about that as a part of future research.

3. Conclusion

In summary, by the second trimester, developmental disorders affecting the nervous system can be diagnosed with a high degree of certainty by ultrasound, but in case of doubtful findings, additional imaging tests should be performed. The development of these disorders is multifactorial; both environmental and genetic factors play a role. In the case of an abnormal ultrasound finding, genetic testing should be performed to confirm the finding and to rule out inherited mutations in subsequent pregnancies.

Author details

Artur Beke*, Virág Bartek and Aténé Simonyi
Department of Obstetrics and Gynecology, Semmelweis University, Budapest, Hungary

*Address all correspondence to: beke.artur@med.semmelweis-univ.hu

References

[1] Chen Z, Kuang L, Finnell RH, Wang H. Genetic and functional analysis of SHROOM1-4 in a Chinese neural tube defect cohort. Human Genetics. 2018;**137**(3):195-202

[2] Colas J-F, Schoenwolf GC. Towards a cellular and molecular understanding of neurulation. Developmental Dynamics. 2001;**221**(2):117-145. DOI: 10.1002/dvdy.1144

[3] Seidahmed MZ, Abdelbasit OB, Shaheed MM, Alhussein KA, Miqdad AM, Khalil MI, et al. Epidemiology of neural tube defects. Saudi Medical Journal. 2014;**35**(Suppl 1):S29-S35

[4] Tafuri SM, Lui F. Embryology, Anencephaly. 2021 May 8. In: StatPearls [Internet]. Treasure Island (FL): StatPearls Publishing; Jan 2022. PMID: 31424828

[5] Papp Z. A szülészet-nőgyógyászat tankönyve. Vol. 4. Budapest, Semmelweis Kiadó; 2009

[6] Horcajadas A, Palma A, Khalon BM. Frontoethmoidal encephalocele. Report of a case. Neurocirugía (Asturias, Spain). 2019;**30**(2):94-99. DOI: 10.1016/j.neucir.2018.02.006

[7] Suwanwela C, Suwanwela N. A morphological classification of sincipital encephalomeningoceles. Journal of Neurosurgery. Feb 1972;**36**(2):201-211. DOI: 10.3171/jns.1972.36.2.0201. PMID: 5008734

[8] Kancherla V, Wagh K, Johnson Q, Oakley GP Jr. A 2017 global update on folic acid-preventable spina bifida and anencephaly. Birth Defects Research. 2018;**110**(14):1139-1147. DOI: 10.1002/bdr1132.1366

[9] Shields DC, Kirke PN, Mills JL, Ramsbottom D, Molloy AM, Burke H, et al. The "thermolabile" variant of methylenetetrahydrofolate reductase and neural tube defects: An evaluation of genetic risk and the relative importance of the genotypes of the embryo and the mother. American Journal of Human Genetics. 1999;**64**(4):1045-1055

[10] McGreevy EM, Vijayraghavan D, Davidson LA, Hildebrand JD. Shroom3 functions downstream of planar cell polarity to regulate myosin II distribution and cellular organization during neural tube closure. Biology Open. 2015;**4**(2):186-196

[11] Murdoch JN, Damrau C, Paudyal A, Bogani D, Wells S, Greene NDE, et al. Genetic interactions between planar cell polarity genes cause diverse neural tube defects in mice. Disease Models & Mechanisms. 2014;**7**(10):1153-1163

[12] Valentin M, Coste Mazeau P, Zerah M, Ceccaldi PF, Benachi A, Luton D. Acid folic and pregnancy: A mandatory supplementation. Annales d'Endocrinologie. 2018;**79**(2):91-94

[13] Avagliano L, Massa V, George TM, Qureshy S, Bulfamante GP, Finnell RH. Overview on neural tube defects: From development to physical characteristics. Birth Defects Research. 2019;**111**(19):1455-1467. DOI: 10.1002/bdr1452.1380

[14] Turhan AH, Isik S. Neural tube defects: A retrospective study of 69 cases. Asian Journal of Neurosurgery. 2019;**14**(2):506-509

[15] Micu R, Chicea AL, Bratu DG, Nita P, Nemeti G, Chicea R. Ultrasound and magnetic resonance imaging in

the prenatal diagnosis of open spina bifida. Medical Ultrasonography. 2018;**20**(2):2018. DOI: 10.11152/mu-1325

[16] Kennedy D, Chitayat D, Winsor EJT, Silver M, Toi A. Prenatally diagnosed neural tube defects: Ultrasound, chromosome, and autopsy or postnatal findings in 212 cases. American Journal of Medical Genetics. 1998;**77**(4):317-321

[17] Wainwright HC. Embryo and Fetal pathology. Color atlas with ultrasound correlation. Journal of Clinical Pathology. 2005;**58**:784. DOI: 10.1136/jcp.2005.026047

[18] D'Antonio F, Zafeiriou DI. Fetal ventriculomegaly: What we have and what is still missing. European Journal of Pediatric Neurology. 2018;**22**(6):898-899. DOI: 10.1016/j.ejpn.2018.11.005

[19] Tully HM, Dobyns WB. Infantile hydrocephalus: A review of epidemiology, classification and causes. Europen Journal of Medical Genetics. 2014;**57**(8):359-368. DOI: 10.1016/j.ejmg.2014.06.002

[20] Saugier-Veber P, Marguet F, Lecoquierre F, Adle-Biassette H, Guimiot F, Cipriani S, et al. Hydrocephalus due to multiple ependymal malformations is caused by mutations in the MPDZ gene. Acta Neuropathologica Communications. 2017;**5**(1):36. DOI: 10.1186/s40478-017-0438-4

[21] Yamasaki M, Nonaka M, Bamba Y, Teramoto C, Ban C, Pooh RK. Diagnosis, treatment, and long-term outcomes of fetal hydrocephalus. Seminars in Fetal and Neonatal Medicine. 2012;**17**(6):330-335. DOI: 10.1016/j.siny.2012.07.004

[22] Fox NS, Monteagudo A, Kuller JA, Craigo S, Norton ME. Mild fetal ventriculomegaly: Diagnosis, evaluation, and management. American Journal of Obstetrics and Gynecology. 2018;**219**(1):B2-B9. DOI: 10.1016/j.ajog.2018.04.039

[23] Shaheen R, Sebai MA, Patel N, Ewida N, Kurdi W, Altweijri I, et al. The genetic landscape of familial congenital hydrocephalus. Annals of Neurology. 2017;**81**(6):890-897. DOI: 10.1002/ana.24964

[24] Assémat E, Crost E, Ponserre M, Wijnholds J, Le Bivic A, Massey-Harroche D. The multi-PDZ domain protein-1 (MUPP-1) expression regulates cellular levels of the PALS-1/PATJ polarity complex. Experimental Cell Research. 2013;**319**(17):2514-2525. DOI: 10.1016/j.yexcr.2013.07.011

[25] Drielsma A, Jalas C, Simonis N, Désir J, Simanovsky N, Pirson I, et al. Two novel CCDC88C mutations confirm the role of DAPLE in autosomal recessive congenital hydrocephalus. Journal of Medical Genetics. 2012;**49**(11):708-712. DOI: 10.1136/jmedgenet-2012-101190

[26] Ishida-Takagishi M, Enomoto A, Asai N, Ushida K, Watanabe T, Hashimoto T, et al. The dishevelled-associating protein Daple controls the non-canonical Wnt/Rac pathway and cell motility. Nature Communications. 2012;**3**:859. DOI: 10.1038/ncomms1861

[27] Blaas HG, Eik-Nes SH. Sonoembryology and early prenatal diagnosis of neural anomalies. Prenatal Diagnosis. 2009;**29**(4):312-325. DOI: 10.1002/pd.2170

[28] Breeze A, Alexander P, Murdoch E, Missfelder-Lobos H, Hackett G, Lees C. Obstetric and neonatal outcome in severe ventriculomegaly. Prenatal Diagnosis. 2007;**27**:124-129. DOI: 10.1002/pd.1624

[29] Pisapia JM, Sinha S, Zarnow DM, Johnson MP, Heuer GG. Fetal ventriculomegaly: Diagnosis, treatment, and future directions. Child's Nervous System. 2017;**33**(7):1113-1123. DOI: 10.1007/s00381-017-3441-y

[30] Kahle KT, Kulkarni AV, Limbrick DD Jr, Warf BC. Hydrocephalus in children. Lancet. 2016;**387**(10020):788-799. DOI: 10.1016/s0140-6736(15)60694-8

[31] Swaiman KF. Swaiman's pediatric neurology: Principles and practice. 6th edition. Edinburgh: Elsevier Saunders; 2012;S199-202

[32] Hunter A, Jimenez C, Tawagi F. Familial renal-hepatic-pancreatic dysplasia and Dandy-Walker cyst: A distinct syndrome? American Journal of Medical Genetics. 1991;**41**(2):201-207

[33] Capra V, Iacomino M, Accogli A, Pavanello M, Zara F, Cama A, et al. Chiari malformation type I: What information from the genetics? Child's Nervous System. 2019;**35**(10):1665-1671. DOI: 10.1007/s00381-019-04322-w

[34] Lieb JM, Ahlhelm FJ. Balkenfehlbildungen. Der Radiologe. 2018;**58**(7):636-645. DOI: 10.1007/s00117-018-0388-2

[35] Palmer EE, Mowat D. Agenesis of the corpus callosum: A clinical approach to diagnosis. American Journal of Medical Genetics. 2014;**166c**(2):184-197. DOI: 10.1002/ajmg.c.31405

[36] Aicardi J. Aicardi syndrome. Brain and Development. 2005;**27**(3):164-171. DOI: 10.1016/j.braindev.2003.11.011

[37] Santo S, D'Antonio F, Homfray T, Rich P, Pilu G, Bhide A, et al. Counseling in fetal medicine: Agenesis of the corpus callosum. Ultrasound in Obstetrics and Gynecology. 2012;**40**(5):513-521. DOI: 10.1002/uog.12315

[38] Ming JE, Muenke M. Multiple hits during early embryonic development: Digenic diseases and holoprosencephaly. American Journal of Human Genetics. 2002;**71**(5):1017-1032. DOI: 10.1086/344412

[39] Tekendo-Ngongang C, Muenke M, Kruszka P. Holoprosencephaly overview. In: Adam MP, Ardinger HH, Pagon RA, Wallace SE, Bean LJH, Stephens K, Amemiya A, editors. GeneReviews(®). Seattle: University of Washington; 1993

[40] Ming JE, Roessler E, Muenke M. Human developmental disorders and the sonic hedgehog pathway. Molecular Medicine Today. 1998;**4**(8):343-349. DOI: 10.1016/s1357-4310(98)01299-4

[41] Cohen MM Jr. Holoprosencephaly: Clinical, anatomic, and molecular dimensions. Birth Defects Research. 2006;**76**(9):658-673. DOI: 10.1002/bdra.20295

[42] Belloni E, Muenke M, Roessler E, Traverso G, Siegel-Bartelt J, Frumkin A, et al. Identification of sonic hedgehog as a candidate gene responsible for holoprosencephaly. Nature Genetics. 1996;**14**(3):353-356. DOI: 10.1038/ng1196-353

[43] Geng X, Speirs C, Lagutin O, Inbal A, Liu W, Solnica-Krezel L, et al. Haploinsufficiency of Six3 fails to activate sonic hedgehog expression in the ventral forebrain and causes holoprosencephaly. Developmental Cell. 2008;**15**(2):236-247. DOI: 10.1016/j.devcel.2008.07.003

[44] Kousa YA, du Plessis AJ, Vezina G. Prenatal diagnosis of holoprosencephaly. American Journal of Medical Genetics Part C: Seminars in Medical Genetics. 2018;**178**(2):206-213. DOI: 10.1002/ajmg.c.31618

[45] Kaliaperumal C, Ndoro S, Mandiwanza T, Reidy F, McAuliffe F,

Caird J, et al. Holoprosencephaly: Antenatal and postnatal diagnosis and outcome. Childs Nervous System. 2016;**32**(5):801-809. DOI: 10.1007/s00381-016-3015-4

[46] Arroyo HA. Microcephaly. Medicina (B Aires). 2018;**78**(Suppl 2):94-100 (Microcefalia.)

[47] Woods CG, Parker A. Investigating microcephaly. Archives of Disease in Childhood. 2013;**98**(9):707-713. DOI: 10.1136/archdischild-2012-302882

[48] Faheem M, Naseer MI, Rasool M, Chaudhary AG, Kumosani TA, Ilyas AM, et al. Molecular genetics of human primary microcephaly: An overview. BMC Medical Genomics. 2015;**8**(Suppl 1(Suppl 1)):S4. DOI: 10.1186/1755-8794-8-s1-s4

[49] de Oliveira WK, de França GVA, Carmo EH, Duncan BB, de Souza Kuchenbecker R, Schmidt MI. Infection-related microcephaly after the 2015 and 2016 Zika virus outbreaks in Brazil: A surveillance-based analysis. Lancet. 2017;**390**(10097):861-870. DOI: 10.1016/s0140-6736(17)31368-5

[50] de Castro M, Doin Trigo LA, Benini-Junior JR, Brito LGO, Marba STM, Amaral E. Ultrasound diagnosis of microcephaly: A comparison of three reference curves and postnatal diagnosis. Archives of Gynecology and Obstetrics. 2019;**300**(5):1211-1219. DOI: 10.1007/s00404-019-05234-5

[51] Bicknell LS, Walker S, Klingseisen A, Stiff T, Leitch A, Kerzendorfer C, et al. Mutations in ORC1, encoding the largest subunit of the origin recognition complex, cause microcephalic primordial dwarfism resembling Meier-Gorlin syndrome. Nature Genetics. 2011;**43**(4):350-355. DOI: 10.1038/ng.776

[52] Alcantara D, O'Driscoll M. Congenital microcephaly. American Journal of Medical Genetics. 2014; **166c**(2):124-139. DOI: 10.1002/ajmg.c.31397

[53] Sadler TW, Langman J. Langman's Medical Embryology. Vol. 1. Philadelphia: Wolters Kluwer Health/Lippincott Williams & Wilkins; 2012. p. c2012

[54] Taguchi T. Sacrococcygeal teratoma: Nationwide survey and guidelines. Pediatrics International. 2019;**61**(7):633. DOI: 10.1111/ped.13933

[55] Graf JL, Albanese CT. Fetal sacrococcygeal teratoma. World Journal of Surgery. 2003;**27**(1):84-86. DOI: 10.1007/s00268-002-6741-6

[56] Kremer MEB, Althof JF, Derikx JPM, van Baren R, Heij HA, Wijnen M, et al. The incidence of associated abnormalities in patients with sacrococcygeal teratoma. Journal of Pediatric Surgery. 2018;**53**(10):1918-1922. DOI: 10.1016/j.jpedsurg.2018.01.013

[57] Dalal SS, Berry T, Pimentel VM. Prenatal Sacrococcygeal Teratoma diagnosed in a Fetus with partial trisomy 13q22. Case Report in Obstetrics and Gynecology. 2019;**2019**:2892869. DOI: 10.1155/2019/2892869

[58] Mylonas KS, Kao CS, Levy D, Lordello L, Dal Cin P, Masiakos PT, et al. Clinicopathologic features and chromosome 12p status of Pediatric Sacrococcygeal Teratomas: A multi-institutional analysis. Pediatric and Development Pathology. 2019;**22**(3):214-220. DOI: 10.1177/1093526618798771

[59] Emerson RE, Kao CS, Eble JN, Grignon DJ, Wang M, Zhang S, et al. Evidence of a dual histogenetic pathway of sacrococcygeal teratomas. Histopathology. 2017;**70**(2):290-300. DOI: 10.1111/his.13062

[60] Emans PJ, Kootstra G, Marcelis CL, Beuls EA, van Heurn LW. The Currarino triad: The variable expression. Journal of Pediatric Surgery. 2005;**40**(8):1238-1242. DOI: 10.1016/j.jpedsurg.2005.05.004

[61] Stroustrup Smith A, Levine D, Barnes PD, Robertson RL. Magnetic resonance imaging of the kinked fetal brain stem: A sign of severe dysgenesis. Journal of Ultrasound in Medicine. 2005;**24**(12):1697-1709. DOI: 10.7863/jum.2005.24.12.1697

[62] Stanislavsky A, Kang O. Kinked brainstem. Reference article, Radiopaedia.org. [Accessed on 25 Mar 2022] DOI: 10.53347/rID-51058

[63] Amir T, Poretti A, Boltshauser E, Huisman TA. Differential diagnosis of ventriculomegaly and brainstem kinking on fetal MRI. Brain Development. 2016;**38**(1):103-108. DOI: 10.1016/j.braindev.2015.05.006

[64] Bönnemann CG, Wang CH, Quijano-Roy S, Deconinck N, Bertini E, Ferreiro A, et al. Diagnostic approach to the congenital muscular dystrophies. Neuromuscular Disorders. 2014;**24**(4):289-311. DOI: 10.1016/j.nmd.2013.12.011

[65] Cabet S, Karl K, Garel C, Delius M, Hartung J, Lesca G, et al. Two different prenatal imaging cerebral patterns of tubulinopathy. Ultrasound in Obstetrics & Gynecology. 2021;**57**(3):493-497. DOI: 10.1002/uog.22010

[66] Chen CP. Prenatal diagnosis of iniencephaly. Taiwanese Journal of Obstetrics and Gynecology. 2007;**46**(3):199-208. DOI: 10.1016/s1028-4559(08)60021-2

[67] Holmes LB, Toufaily MH, Westgate MN. Iniencephaly. Birth Defects Research. 2018;**110**(2):128-133. DOI: 10.1002/bdr2.1082

[68] Tanriverdi EC, Delibas IB, Kamalak Z, Kadioglu BG, Bender RA. A Fetus with Iniencephaly delivered at the third trimester. Case Report in Medicine. 2015;**2015**:520715. DOI: 10.1155/2015/520715

[69] Cuillier F, Koenig P, Lagarde L, Cartault JF. Transvaginal sonographic diagnosis of iniencephaly apertus and craniorachischisis at 9 weeks' gestation. Ultrasound in Obstetrics and Gynecology. 2003;**22**(6):657-658. DOI: 10.1002/uog.895

[70] Greene ND, Stanier P, Moore GE. The emerging role of epigenetic mechanisms in the etiology of neural tube defects. Epigenetics. 2011;**6**(7):875-883. DOI: 10.4161/epi.6.7.16400

[71] Wilde JJ, Petersen JR, Niswander L. Genetic, epigenetic, and environmental contributions to neural tube closure. Annual Reviews of Genetics. 2014;**48**:583-611. DOI: 10.1146/annurev-genet-120213-092208

Chapter 8

Open Fetal Surgery and Fetoscopic Repair in Spina Bifida and Myelomeningocele in Romania

Hadi Rahimian, Ramona Ana Maria Rahimian and Radu Vladareanu

Abstract

Spina bifida and myelomeningocele, although frequent, present difficulties when it comes to diagnosis and clinical management. The recent developments in ultrasound and MRI technologies and software, allow for an easier and more precise diagnosis. As such, in the first part of our chapter we will present general information, such as etiology, pathophysiology and methods of diagnosis. Fetal surgery, open or fetoscopic, represents a cure in most cases of spina bifida and in other cases reduces the chances of major developmental issues in babies born with this affliction. In the second part of our chapter, we will present the surgical protocols for both procedures, the indications, and the statistics that we have acquired in the cases we have diagnosed and operated on in the Regina Maria Maternity Hospital, Bucharest, the only center in Romania where these procedures are available.

Keywords: Spina bifida, Myelomeningocele, Open fetal surgery, Fetoscopic surgery, Fetal prognosis

1. Introduction

Spinal cord defects appear because of failure in the closure of the neural folds. These defects usually appear during the third and fourth weeks of gestation. Neural tube defects (NTD) can affect the meninges, vertebrae, muscles, and the skin. ([1]—Langman's). Meningocele and myelomeningocele are the most frequently encountered spinal dysraphisms.

Closed spinal defects include spina bifida occulta, lipomyelomeingocele and a multitude of other conditions.

Open spinal dysraphisms are mostly compatible with survival but usually the quality of life of the patient will be affected, depending on the level of the aperture. Symptoms are comprised of inability to walk, incontinence, scoliosis, digestive disorders, and hydrocephalus [1, 2].

2. Embryology

Spinal dysraphisms appear from a failure of either: gastrulation, primary neurulation, disjunction or secondary neurulation.

Gastrulation is the process where the bilaminar embryonic disc becomes trilaminar. When this process happens, the neuroenteric canal forms and creates a temporary connection between the dorsal and ventral surface of the trilamiar disc. It is thought that split cord malformations and neuroenteric cysts arise from the persistence of this canal.

Neurulation begins when the formation of the central nervous system by signaling the ectoderm to differentiate and form the neural plate. This plate folds inwards, it's edges connecting to one another, completing the process known as primary neurulation.

After the primary neurulation, the neural tube separates form the ectodermic tissue, this process is known as disjunction. During this process, the mesoderm moves between the ectoderm and the neural tube, creating the meninges, skull, vertebrae and the paraspinal muscles. If this process starts prematurely or it is incomplete, a lypomeningocele or a dermal sinus may form [1].

The secondary neurulation is the formation of the spinal cord above the midsacrum.

Open spinal defects appear from the delay or cessation of the primary neurulation.

Defects during the second neurulation are believed to be the cause for closed spinal dysraphisms.

Signaling pathways and cellular functions are also included in the formation of neural tube defects; planar cell polarity signaling, sonic hedgehog signaling, retinoid signaling and many others are though to be factors.

Some genetic factors, as well as environment factors are also included as rick factors of developing spinal dysraphisms, such as: valproic acid, fungal products (fumonisin), carbamazepine, trimethoprim, and folate and vitamin B12 deficiency, inositol, and maternal diabetes mellitus (environmental factors), the genetic factors include C67TT and a1298C polymorphisms of the methylenetetrahydrofolate reductase, this results in a 1.8-fold increase in risk of NTDs [2, 3].

3. Clinical diagnosis

All pregnancies are at risk for neural tube defects, as such all women of fertile age as well as all pregnant women are encouraged to take folic acid supplements. It is paramount to take a full maternal history, as women with a history of anticonvulsant medication, diabetes or obesity are at higher risk for neural tube defects.

Prenatal clinical diagnosis relies on maternal elevated alpha-fetoprotein levels and amniocentesis, usually performed after 15–16 weeks of gestation. Although an early amniocentesis can be performed between 10 and 14 weeks of gestation, the low quantity amniotic fluid at this gestational age forces the practitioner to withdraw a smaller quantity which may not provide enough cells for analysis.

In the case of neural tube defects, an elevated alpha-fetoprotein and acetylcholinesterase level in the amniotic fluid and maternal blood usually prompts further investigations, such as high-resolution fetal ultrasonography and MRI [3, 4].

4. Imaging

4.1 Ultrasound

Identifying spinal anomalies during a routine ultrasound screening usually varies depending on the skill and expertise of the operator.

A very detailed protocol should be followed for a correct diagnosis, both axial and longitudinal views of the spine have to be obtained. It is important to know the precise timing of ossification for each segment of spine. At 16 weeks ossification is complete up to L5, by 19 weeks it reaches S1 and by 22 weeks the process is complete. The best plane for the visualization of everted pedicles is the transverse one, as for an overlying sac, both transverse and longitudinal planes should be used as well as a high frequency transducer that would show cord tethering or placode content (**Figures 1** and **2**).

Chiari II malformations are very often encountered in fetuses with neural tube defects so, it is paramount that the fetal brain is scanned initially. Findings such as a small cisterna magna along with a rounded cerebellum (banana sign), concaved frontal bones (lemon sign) and ventriculomegaly are suggestive for Chiari II malformation. The banana sign has a 99% sensitivity in the diagnostic, the lemon sign has a lower sensitivity rate and can be present in normal fetuses [5].

4.2 MRI

The MRI has become an invaluable addition in the diagnosis and preoperative preparation of spinal dysraphisms. 1.5 Tesla magnets are usually used although a 3 Tesla magnet can be useful in maximizing image quality. Orthogonal planes can also be used, adjusted to the preceding image set if the fetal position changes (**Figure 3**).

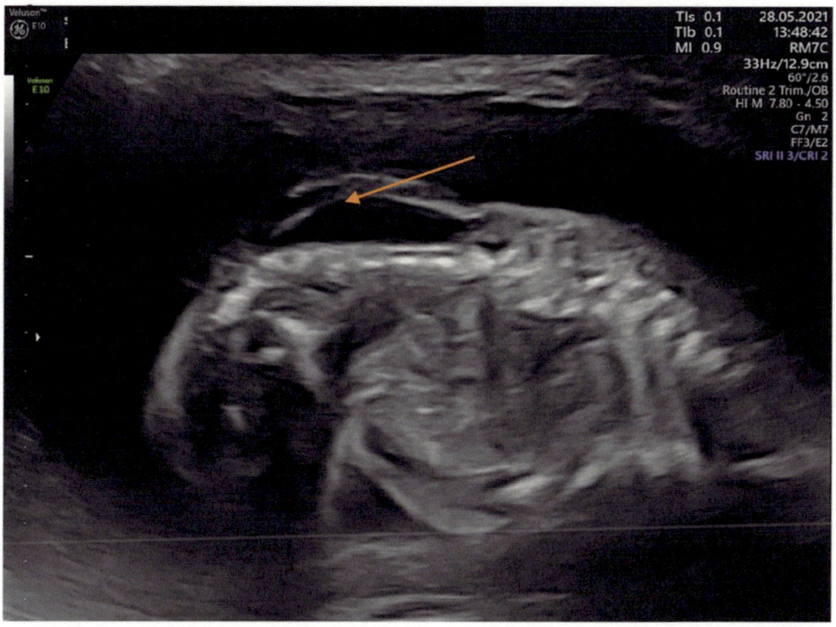

Figure 1.
Ultrasound depiction of a spinal dysraphism (arrow) during a routine 2nd trimester examination.

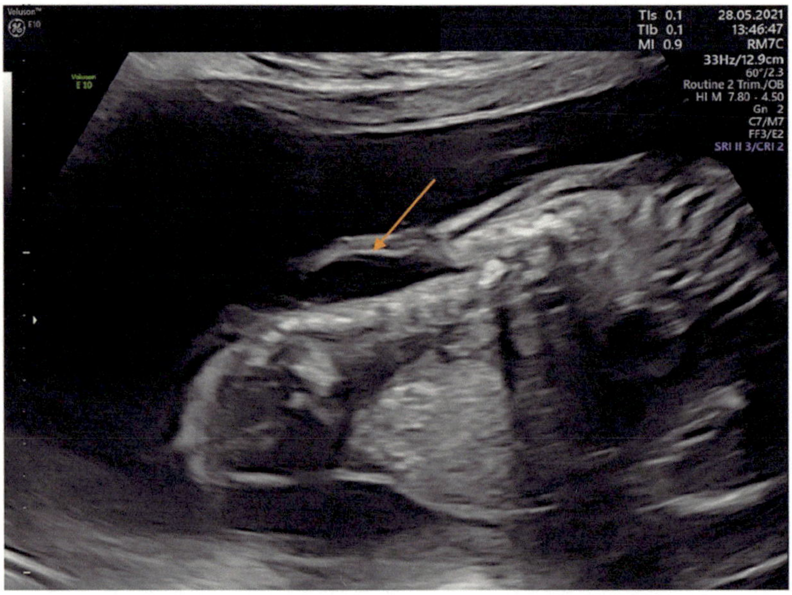

Figure 2.
Ultrasound picture (same case as **Figure 1***) in a different position where it is shown that there is no cord tethering (arrow).*

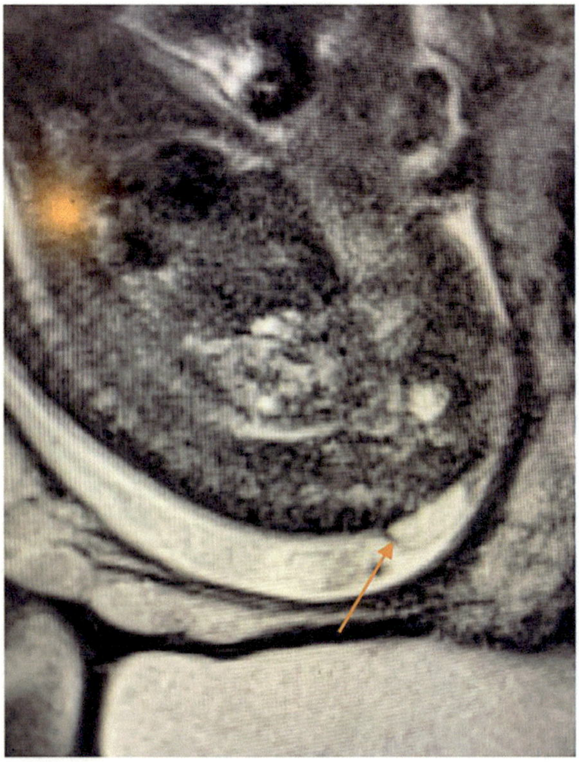

Figure 3.
MRI imaging of large, closed spina bifida defect (arrow).

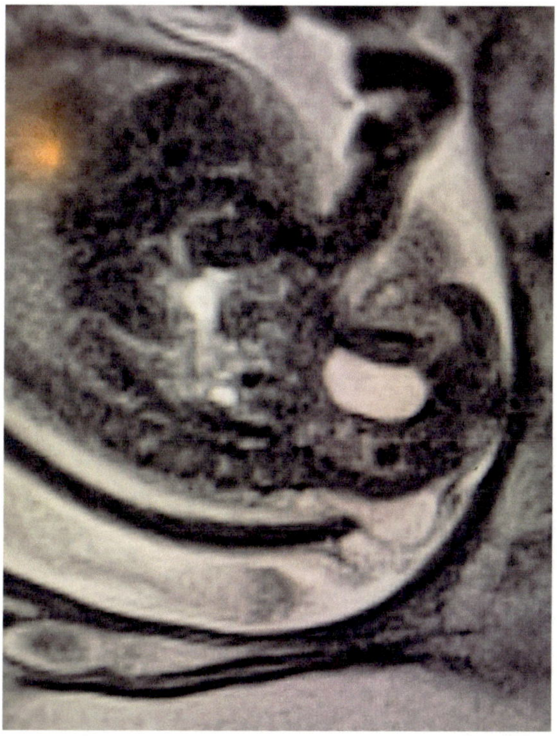

Figure 4.
MRI imaging showing closed neural tube defect (arrow).

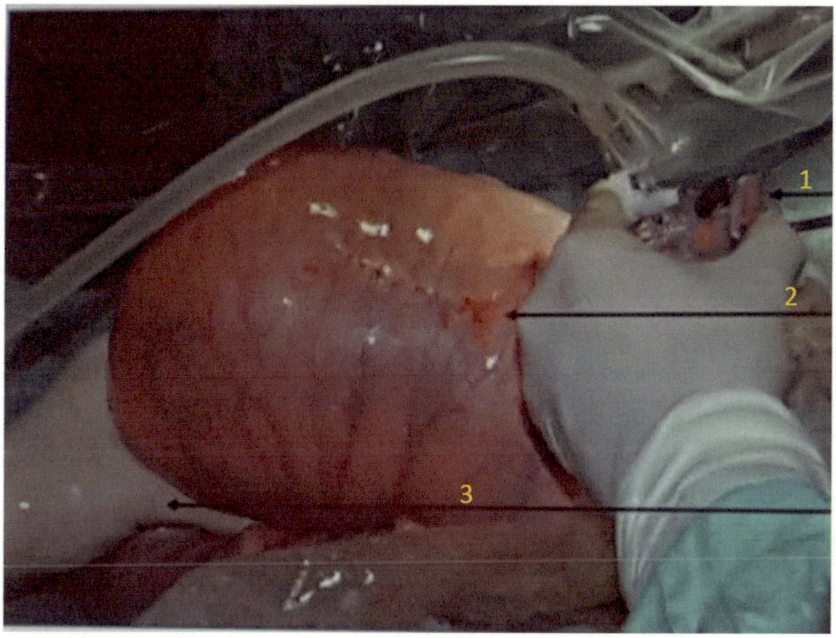

Figure 5.
1. Placement of fetoscopic trocars 2. Uterine wall 3. One hand is holding the fetus in order to create the pocket of gas in front of the operating field.

In order to pinpoint the fetal position a localizer sequence has to be used to guide the initial imaging plane which is aligned with the fetal anatomy that has to be examined. Ultrafast sequencing can also be used to minimize image degradation by fetal movements (**Figure 3**).

Single shot fast spin echo or half-Fourier acquisition single-shot fast spin echo sequences at 2 to 4 mm slice thickness are used to provide most of the diagnostic information (**Figure 4**) [6].

5. Treatment

5.1 Fetal surgery

5.1.1 History of spina bifida surgeries

The first time a spina bifida repair was performed was in 1994 using an endoscopic technique. In 1997 the first open(hysterotomy) in-utero spina bifida repair was performed at Vanderbilt University and at The Children's Hospital of Philadelphia.

The experience of these institutions suggested that babies treated in utero had a decreased incidence of hindbrain herniation and that after three weeks post-intervention, the hindbrain structures would ascent. Chiari II malformations were improved whereas other Chiari modifications were not (such as thinning of the corpus callosum), however it was shortly proven that the placement of fetal shunts is unnecessary in most cases.

The follow up also showed that after fetal surgery was performed the number of patients needing shut placement after birth has decreased significantly. Although most infants did not require shunting in the newborn period, some required it within the first year of life. A comparison between patients that underwent the fetal procedure prior to 26 weeks of gestation and those after 25 weeks of gestation showed that early fetal closure eliminates the leakage of spinal fluid and creates a back-pressure, reducing the herniation of the hindbrain.

Because of the selection and short follow-up processes in these cases, it was difficult to demonstrate the benefit to lower extremity function and sphincter continence, as well as cognitive function. However, findings showed an improved healing and scar formation, resulting in a more esthetic result [7, 8].

5.1.2 Surgical technique

The decision to perform fetal surgery for spina bifida relies on the inclusion and exclusion criteria established in the world renown MOMS study (**Table 1**). To make a correct and informed decision, a high-resolution fetal ultrasonography, a fetal MRI scan as well as maternal and fetal serology are necessary in order to assess the extent of the defect. In any fetal operation maternal safety comes first, after which the next major goal is avoiding preterm labor. Spinal dysraphism repairs should be performed between 18 and 27 weeks of gestation, prior to this interval the fetal size would be too small and the tissues too fragile to accommodate the intervention and after 27 weeks of gestation there would be no shown benefit to the surgery compared to post-natal repair (**Table 1**).

This surgery requires a team that includes maternal-fetal specialists, neurosurgeons, pediatric surgeons, neonatologists, radiologists, anesthesiologists, and

Inclusion Criteria:
Myelomeningocele at level T1-S1 with hindbrain herniation
Maternal age > 18 years
Gestational age between 18 and 25 weeks of gestation usually measured according to the first ultrasound and not patient's last menstrual period
Normal karyotype with written confirmation of culture results
Exclusion criteria:
Multifetal pregnancy
Abnormal foetal echocardiogram
Other related/unrelated foetal anomalies
Documented history of incompetent cervix
Cervix <20 mm measured by ultrasound
Preterm labour in current pregnancy
History of recurrent preterm labour
Maternal-foetal Rh isoimmunisation, Kell sensitisation, history of neonatal alloimmune thrombocytopenia
Maternal HIV or hepatitis B status positive or unknown
Uterine anomalies
Maternal medical conditions that are a contraindication to surgery or anesthesia
Maternal obesity
Placenta praevia
Fetal kyphosis >30°

Table 1.
Inclusion and exclusion criteria according to MOMS (Management of Myelomeningocele study) [7].

geneticists. The mother should always receive counseling and all the team members should explain their roles in detail before the procedure [7].

Drug therapy to decrease the chances of preterm labor should be administered as follows: magnesium sulfate preoperatively and for the first 18–48 hours following surgery, indomethacin preoperatively and continued for 48 hours, oral nifedipine preoperatively and continued until delivery and terbutaline sulfate administered subcutaneously continuously by a pump if the other medication fails.

Anesthesia in neural dysraphism repairs is particularly complex as it affects both mother and fetus and it must take in consideration the uteroplacental factor. An epidural catheter is placed for postoperative analgesia before the rapid sequence induction and the intubation are performed. Desflurane is usually used for maintaining the anesthesia, but nitrous oxide can also be a choice. Tice the amount of alveolar concentration is usually used to achieve uterine relaxation. In order to keep the arterial blood pressure close to the pre-induction base-line, ephedrine or phenylephrine is used. Vecuronium is administered for neuromuscular blockade.

The fetus also must be anesthetized before incision, usually with a narcotic and a muscle blocker delivered intramuscularly [9].

There are three possible methods of performing spina bifida fetal interventions: open surgery, fetoscopy procedure and endoscopically (abandoned as it presented a high risk of membrane rupture and was proved unsatisfactory compared to the other two methods).

For open surgery, the uterus is exposed though a low transverse abdominal incision, using ultrasonography the fetal and placental positions are determined and the uterus is placed to have proper exposure. Hemostatic sutures are applied where the future incision will be, then with a monopolar cautery the hysterotomy is performed between these sutures. The incision is enlarged using a stapler that simultaneously cuts the uterine wall as well as applies hemostatic absorbable clips that will hold the amniotic membranes (**Figures 6** and 7). Because the incision is in the upper portion of the uterine segment, it is important to relate to the mother that this and any future pregnancies will have to be delivered by C-section.

Maintaining uterine volume is paramount as it prevents placental separation, contractions, and fetal expulsion. For this reason, warm Ringer lactate solution is continuously pumped into the uterine cavity and the fetus is not completely removed from the cavity, only being moved as much as needed to get optimal access to the operating area (**Figure 8**).

The myelomeningocele is closed rapidly and with as little blood loss as possible, the technique being similar to the standard post-natal variant. The full-thickness skin is incised circumferentially with a 15-blade knife until it reaches the fascia, the sac is mobilized to the facial defect, it is excised from the placode, removing all epithelial tissue

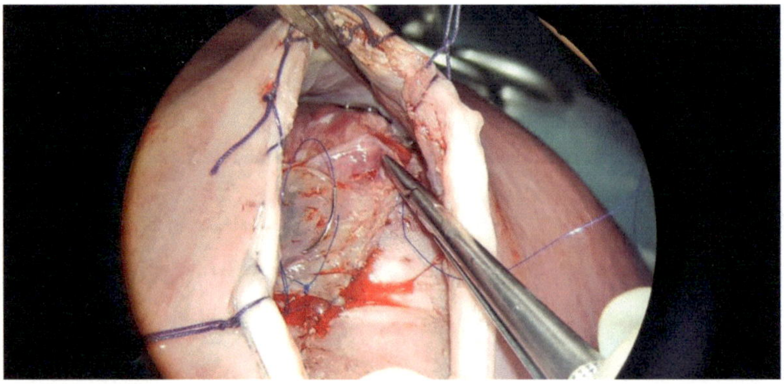

Figure 6.
Microscopic view of open spina bifida surgery. The amniotic membranes are sutured to the uterine wall. The defect is visible (arow) and our neurosurgeon started the repair.

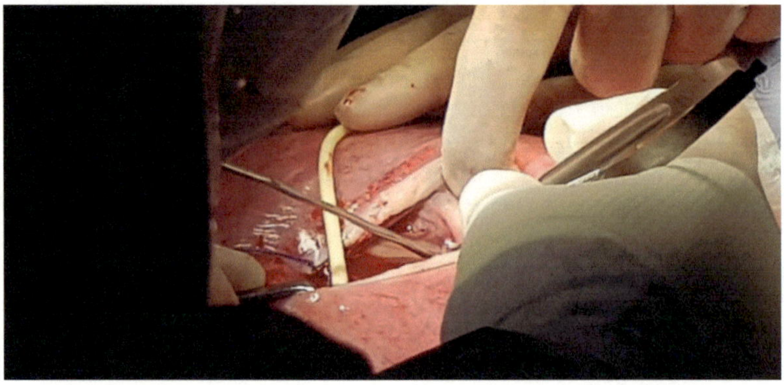

Figure 7.
Open spina bifida surgery. The Folley catheter is used to insert warm saline solution in the uterine cavity to replenish the lost amniotic fluid.

in order to prevent future epidermoid inclusion cyst formation. The re-neurulation of the placode is not attempted as at this gestational age the tissues are extremely friable. It is preferred that the closure be done with dura and undermined fascia but either dura or fascia alone can lead to a successful result (**Figure 9**). The skin is closed with a 4–0 absorbable PDA suture, if the defect is too large acellular human graft material can be used.

The uterus is closed with a tight two-layer closure and transparent dressing must be used in order to perform future ultrasonographic examinations [7].

The fetoscopic procedure begins as well with a transverse abdominal incision but this time the uterus is taken out of the abdominal cavity. Two or three ports are inserted in the uterine cavity through small incisions, under ultrasonographic guidance (**Figure 5**). A small quantity of amniotic fluid is taken out and replaced with CO2 to have a better visualization. It is very important that before the repair is commenced that a narcotic injection is administered to the fetus in order to have

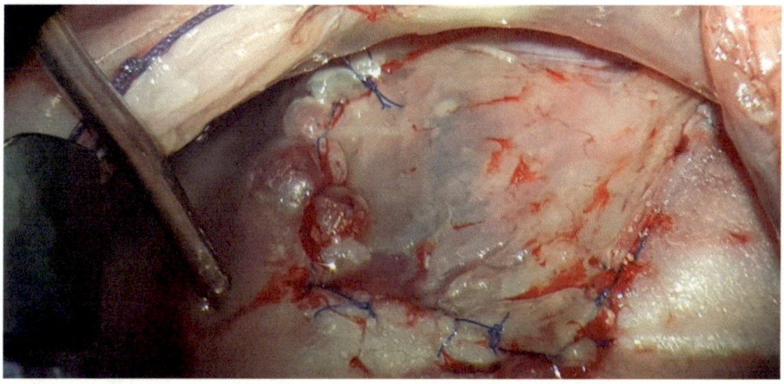

Figure 8.
Open spina bifida surgery. Final aspect of the repaired site (arrow).

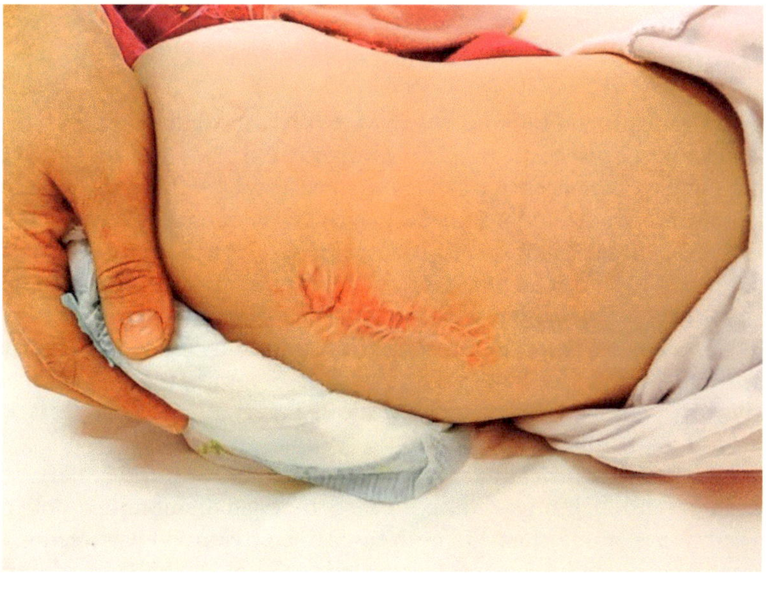

Figure 9.
Open spina bifida surgery. 1 month post-natal aspect of the surgery site.

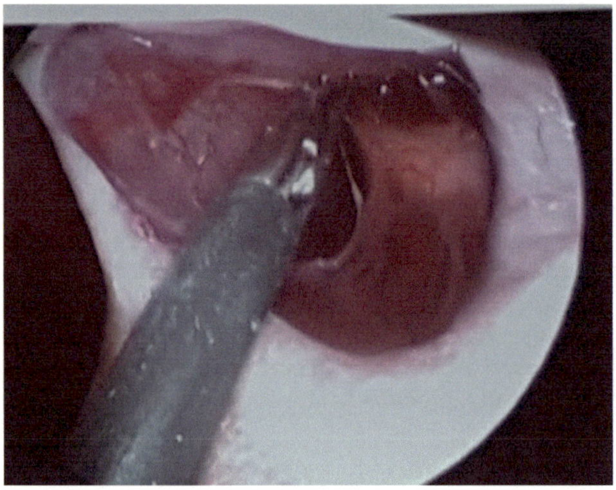

Figure 10.
Fetoscopic view of myelomeningocele defect before repair.

analgesia. The myelomeningocele sac is reduced by the neurosurgeon and the defect is then sutured. In the case of fetoscopic surgery, grafting is not possible as the trocar size does not permit it's passing so the extent of the defect must be meticulously asserted before the procedure (**Figure 10**).

Recent studies have shown that the fetoscopic procedure leads to equal success rates and better post-operative results when it comes to scarring compared to the open surgery. Also, future pregnancies can be delivered vaginally as the uterine scarring is minimal. Fetal short term neurosurgical results are similar to the open fetal surgery, 70% hindbrain herniation ascent and 45% of the patients did not need future treatment for hydrocephaly. The fetoscopic approach minimizes the risk of membrane ruptures and preterm delivery.

5.2 Statistics in our materno-fetal surgical center

In our materno-fetal center Regina Maria Maternity Hospital Baneasa we had a total of 37 patients whose fetuses were diagnosed with spina bifida between 2011 and 2021. Out of these 8 did not have the necessary inclusion criteria and 4 refused the intervention.

At the beginnings we started performing exclusively open surgeries. In total we have performed 18 open surgeries for spina bifida defects, out of these 6 gave birth before 30 weeks of gestation, 5 after 30 weeks of gestation and 7 after 34 weeks of gestation.

As the technology evolved and we have become more proficient in solving these cases, we have decided to perform fetoscopic interventions for spina bifida aswell. As such, from 2011 until 2021 we have performed 8 fetoscopic surgeries. In these cases, 1 patient gave birth before 30 weeks of gestation, 2 after 30 weeks of gestation and 5 after 35 weeks of gestation.

We did not have to perform any emergency hysterectomies during or after the spina bifida defect intervention, but we did have 2 cases that had membrane decollation. The decollation was minor (under 1 cm) in both cases so no treatment was needed.

At the one-year follow-up, we have observed that 6 of the babies had motor function impairment and 3 presented with urinary incontinence. Only 6 out of the 26 patients needed surgery for ventriculomegaly performed after birth.

According to our statistics we had a better outcome using the fetoscopic surgical method for spina bifida as the cases of birth under 30 weeks of gestation were significantly lower compared to open surgery. The results for after 30 weeks of gestation and after 34 weeks of gestation are comparable between the open and the fetosopic spina bifida repairment methods (**Table 2**).

Compared to the 2019 Zurich Center for Fetal Diagnosis and Therapy and the MOMS trial, our center delivers comparable results as seen in **Tables 3** and **4**. Even though the number of patients is not an exact match to the MOMS trial, it is comparable to the Zurich study (**Table 3**) [10].

Our values show a diminished rate of maternal complications compared to the MOMS trial, the only prenatal complication encountered was chorioamniotic membrane separation. The hysterotomy site at delivery was intact in 77% of the cases, 20% very thin, 0% had an area of dehiscence and 3% complete dehiscence. Compared to the Zurich study, we showed a higher rate of well-healed hysterotomy site (77% vs. 40%) but a higher rate of complete dehiscence (3% vs. 0%) (**Table 4**).

Our fetal and neonatal outcomes show that compared to the Zurich trial the percentage of apnea and foot deformity is much higher, however when compared to the MOMS trial we show a much lower rate for these complications.

	Open fetal surgery	Fetoscopic surgery	Total number of cases
No. of cases	18	8	26
<30 weeks of gestation	33.33%	12.50%	26.92%
>30 weeks of gestation	27.77%	25%	26.92%
>34 weeks of gestation	46.15%	46.15%	46.15%

Table 2.
Percentages of births according to weeks of gestation and surgical method.

	MOMS	Zurich	Regina Maria Maternity Hospital Bucharest
Components of the primary outcome, n (%)			
Death before shunt placement	2 (3)	1 (5)	0 (0)
Shunt criteria met	51 (65)	11 (55)	15 (60)
Shunt placed without meeting criteria	0	0	0
Degree of hindbrain herniation			
None	25/70 (36)	17/18 (94)	7/26 (26)
Mild	28/70 (40)	1/18 (6)	10/26 (40)
Moderate	13/70 (36)	0/18 (0)	9/26 (34)
Severe	0 (0)	0 (0)	0 (0)

Table 3.
Infant outcome at 12 months (table modified from Zurich Center data).

	MOMS (n = 78)	Zurich (n = 20)	Regina Maria Maternity Bucharest (n = 26)
Maternal outcome			
Chorioamniotic membrane separation, n (%)	20 (26)	5 (25)	2 (7)
Pulmonary edema, n (%)	5 (6)	0 (0)	0 (0)
Oligohydramnios, n (%)	16 (21)	4 (20)	0 (0)
Placental abruption, n (%)	5 (6)	0 (0)	0 (0)
Gestational diabetes, n (%)	4 (5)	3 (15)	0 (0)
Chorioamniotitis, n (%)	2 (3)	0 (0)	0 (0)
Preeclampsia or gestational hypertension, n (%)	3 (4)	0 (0)	0 (0)
Spontaneous labour, n (%)	30 (38)	13 (65)	0 (0)
Blood transfusion at delivery, n (%)	7 (9)	0 (0)	0 (0)
Status of hysterotomy site at delivery, n/total n (%)			
Intact, well-healed	46/76 (64)	8/20 (40)	20/26 (77)
Very thin	19/76 (25)	10/20 (50)	5/26 (20)
Area of dehiscence	7/76 (9)	2/20 (10)	0/26 (0)
Complete dehiscence	1/76 (1)	0/20 (0)	1/26 (3)
Fetal or neonatal outcome			
Bradycardia during fetal repair, n (%)	8 (10)	1 (5)	4 (15)
Perinatal death, n (%)	2 (3)	1 (5)	0 (0)
Apnea, n/total n (%)	28/77 (36)	1/20 (5)	5/26 (20)
Pneumothorax, n/total n (%)	1/77 (1)	1/20 (5)	0/26 (0)
Respiratory distress syndrome, n/total n (%)	16/77 (21)	7/20 (35)	5/26 (20)
Patent ductus arteriosus, n/total n (%)	3/77 (4)	0/20 (0)	0 (0)
Sepsis, n/total n (%)	4/77 (5)	1/19 (5)	0 (0)
Necrotizing enterocolitis, n/total n (%)	1/77 (1)	0/19 (0)	0 (0)
Periventricular leukomalacia, n/total n (%)	4/77 (5)	0/20 (0)	1/26 (1)
Foot deformity, n/total n (%)	39/78 (50)	5/20 (25)	10/26 (40)

Table 4.
Maternal outcome and fetal or neonatal outcome (table modified from Zurich data Center).

6. Conclusions

Spina bifida is a spinal dysraphism that has a higher incidence compared to other fetal malformations. Fetal surgery for this defect can restore some if not all the sequelae from hindbrain herniation to incontinence giving back the quality of life to the fetus, thus performing the intervention when the criteria are met is necessary especially since the statistic results are positive.

Author details

Hadi Rahimian[1], Ramona Ana Maria Rahimian[2] and Radu Vladareanu[3*]

1 Regina Maria Maternity Hospital, Bucharest, Romania

2 Emergency University Hospital Elias, Bucharest, Romania

3 Carol Davila University of Medicine and Pharmacy, Emergency University Hospital Elias, Bucharest, Romania

*Address all correspondence to: vladareanu@gmail.com

References

[1] Langman's Medical Embryology – 12th edition / T.W. Sadler, ISBN 978-1-4511-1342-6

[2] Fanaroff and Martin's Neonatal-Perinatal Medicine, 2-Volume Set, 11th Edition, ISBN 9780323567114:

[3] McComb JG. A practical clinical classification of spinal neural tube defects. Childs Nerv Syst. 2015;31(10):1641-1657

[4] Klaus and Fanaroff's Care of the High-Risk Neonate, 7th edition, ISBN 978-0-323-60854-1: 409-436

[5] Callen's Ultrasonography in Obstetrics and Gynecology 6th Edition, 2016, ISBN 9780323328340:

[6] Obstetric Imaging: Fetal Diagnosis and Care 2nd Edition, 2017, ISBN 9780323445481: 213-226

[7] Fetal Therapy, Cambridge University Press, 2020, ISBN 9781108564434

[8] Moldenhauer JS, Soni S, Rintoul NE, Spinner SS, Khalek N, Martinez-Poyer J, et al. Fetal myelomeningocele repair: the post-MOMS experience at the Children's Hospital of Philadelphia. Fetal Diagn Ther. 2015; 37(3): 235-240.

[9] Ochsenbein-Kölble N, Krähenmann F, Hüsler M, Meuli M, Moehrlen U, MazzoneL, et al. Tocolysis for in utero surgery: atosiban performs distinctly better than magnesium sulfate. Fetal Diagn Ther. 2018; 44(1): 59-64.

[10] Benchmarking against the MOMS Trial: Zurich Results of Open Fetal Surgery for Spina Bifida, Fetal Diagn Ther 2020;47:91-97, DOI: 10.1159/000500049

Section 3

Prenatal Diagnosis and Screening

Chapter 9

Prenatal Diagnosis: The Main Advances in the Application of Identification of Biomarkers Based on Multi-Omics

Tong Wang, Jiahe Xu, Lin Wang, Xiumin Cui, Yan Yan, Qiuqin Tang and Wei Wu

Abstract

Prenatal diagnosis is to make the diagnosis of fetal structural abnormalities, genetic diseases, and pregnancy-related diseases before birth thus could offer evidence for intrauterine treatment or selectively termination of pregnancy. Up to now, researchers have applied multi-omics, including genomics, transcriptomics, and proteomics, in the discovery of prenatal diagnostic biomarkers. They have found some candidate biomarkers for aneuploids, preeclampsia, intrauterine growth retardation, and congenital structural abnormalities. With the momentous progress of biomarkers' identification based on multi-omics for prenatal diagnosis, noninvasive prenatal testing (NIPT) has experienced tremendous progress and is revolutionizing prenatal screening and diagnosis over the past few decades. Extensive studies have also demonstrated the value of biomarkers. In particular, cell-free DNA (cfDNA), allows for a definitive diagnosis in early pregnancy for fetal diseases, including Down syndrome and other common aneuploidies. The cfDNA can be extracted from maternal plasma, posing no risk of miscarriage compared to the traditional invasive diagnosis directly analyzing fetal cells from amniocentesis or chorionic villus sampling. In this review, we would discuss the main advances, strengths, and limitations in the application of biomarkers for prenatal diagnosis along with the analysis of several representative fetal diseases.

Keywords: aneuploids, biomarker, cell-free DNA, congenital structural abnormalities, intrauterine growth retardation, preeclampsia, prenatal diagnosis

1. Introduction

Prenatal diagnosis is to make the diagnosis of fetal structural abnormalities, genetic diseases, and pregnancy-related diseases before birth thus could offer evidence for intrauterine treatment or selectively termination of pregnancy [1]. Up to now, the research on noninvasive prenatal screening and diagnosis has undergone enormous progress. Researchers around the world have applied multi-omics, including genomics, transcriptomics, and proteomics, in the discovery of prenatal diagnostic biomarkers, and found some candidate biomarkers for aneuploids, pre-eclampsia, intrauterine growth retardation, and congenital structural abnormalities. With the momentous progress of biomarkers' identification based on multi-omics for prenatal diagnosis, noninvasive prenatal testing (NIPT) has made great strides over the past few decades and is revolutionizing prenatal screening and diagnosis. Extensive studies have also demonstrated the value of biomarkers. In particular, cell-free DNA (cfDNA), which is widely acknowledged as the main method of NIPT, allows for a definitive diagnosis in early pregnancy for fetal diseases, including Down syndrome and other common aneuploidies, and thus is sought by providers and patients. In this review, we would discuss the main advances, strengths, and limitations in the application of biomarkers for prenatal diagnosis along with the analysis of several representative fetal diseases.

2. Prenatal diagnostic techniques

2.1 Noninvasive techniques

Noninvasive techniques include examining a woman's uterus through maternal serology and ultrasound. Blood tests for selecting trisomies based on detecting placental cfDNA present in maternal blood, which is also known as NIPT, have now become available [2]. However, if a noninvasive screening test indicates an elevated risk of chromosomal or genetic abnormalities, then invasive techniques can be used to gather more information [3]. For example, a detailed ultrasound can provide a definitive diagnosis noninvasively in the case of neural tube defects (NTDs). Biomarkers are involved in some methods, including maternal serum screening and other methods (**Table 1**).

2.1.1 Fetal cells in maternal blood

The inspection of fetal cells in maternal blood requires a maternal blood draw. Because fetal cells contain nearly all of the genetic information of the developing fetus, they could be used for prenatal diagnosis [4].

2.1.2 Cell-free fetal DNA (cffDNA) in maternal blood

Fetal DNA ranges from about 2–10% of the total DNA in maternal blood. The inspection of cffDNA in maternal blood also requires a maternal blood draw. This test can potentially identify fetal aneuploidy [5] and gender. The cffDNA also allows whole genome sequencing of the fetus, thus determining the complete DNA sequence of every gene [6], which is helpful for prenatal diagnosis.

2.1.3 Transcervical retrieval of trophoblast cells

Cervical swabs, cervical mucus aspiration, and cervical or intrauterine lavage could be used to retrieve trophoblast cells for identifying aneuploidies [7]. It has been proven that antibody markers are available to select trophoblast cells for genetic

i. **Noninvasive techniques:**
• Preimplantation genetic diagnosis (PGD)
• External examination
• Ultrasound detection
• Fetal heartbeat
• Non-stress test
• Maternal blood pressure
• Maternal weighing
• Fetal cells in maternal blood (FCMB)
• Cell-free DNA in maternal blood (cfDNA)
• Glucose tolerance testing
• Transcervical retrieval of trophoblast cells
• Maternal serum screening
ii. **Invasive techniques:**
• Chorionic villus sampling (CVS)
• Amniocentesis
• Embryoscopy and fetoscopy
• Percutaneous umbilical cord blood sampling

Table 1.
Prenatal diagnostic/screening techniques.

analysis or to demonstrate that the abundance of recoverable trophoblast cells is reduced in unusual gestations [7].

2.1.4 Maternal serum screening

Maternal serum screening could be used as a routine prenatal test to determine the risk of aneuploidies as well as certain malformations, including NTDs [8, 9]. Maternal serum screening was classically done in the second trimester but now first-trimester screening has also been found equally useful [8]. The related biomarkers contain β-human chorionic gonadotropin (β-hCG), pregnancy-associated plasma protein-A (PAPP-A), alpha-fetoprotein, and inhibin-A.

2.2 Invasive techniques

An invasive method involves probes or needles being inserted into the uterus. The commonly used invasive methods include amniocentesis and chorionic villus sampling (CVS) [8]. One study has compared second-trimester amniocentesis with transabdominal CVS, finding no significant differences in total pregnancy loss between the two procedures [10]. The samples could be used for molecular, cytogenetic, and biochemical tests but especially, the CVS sample is a perfect sample for DNA-based tests when amniotic fluid is desired for cytogenetic analysis [8].

3. The research of biomarkers based on multi-omics

3.1 Genomics

According to the National Cancer Institute, a biomarker is "a biological molecule which is a sign of normal process or disease found in blood, other body fluids or tissues." Liquid biopsy is very promising for noninvasive characteristics and may provide important biomarkers, including cell-free nucleic acids (cf-NAs) [10]. Since the discovery of free fetal DNA, noninvasive prenatal diagnosis (NIPD) has been gaining attention for early pregnancy detection of genetic diseases by analyzing cfDNA or cffDNA in maternal plasma [11].

First detected in cancer patients' sera in 1948 [12], cfDNA, used as a prognostic factor in malignant disease [9, 13], has gradually shown some advantages in the application of prenatal diagnosis since Lo et al. detected circulating fetal DNA in maternal plasma in 1997 [9, 14]. With the rapid advances in molecular biological technologies, it creates a preferable procedure for chromosomal abnormalities and monogenic disorders. The cfDNA refers to a DNA molecule in plasma, typically between 500 and 30,000 bp nucleotides in size. Existing in peripheral blood, synovial fluid, and other body fluids, cfDNA has three forms—free, attached to proteins, or encapsulated in extracellular vesicles [10]. Based on comprehensive studies, nucleosome spacing of cfDNA in healthy individuals suggests its origin—nucleic or mitochondrial from the apoptosis of lymphoid and myeloid cells [15], mainly swallowed by phagocytes for homeostasis. However, there is no hard evidence to support the origin theory, and the mechanism is not clear. Healthy individuals have less cfDNA. Fetal DNA in maternal circulation (3–6%) is reported to be from placental apoptosis [16].

Using cfDNA as a biomarker is advantageous for the accessible sample with little trauma, dynamic monitoring from early pregnancy, sensitive and specific procedure, and reliable outcome. However, the unit cost of cfDNA is relatively more expensive than invasive tests. Screening for trisomies by cfDNA could detect nearly 100% of fetuses with trisomy 21, 98% of trisomy 18, and 99% of trisomy 13, with a combined false-positive rate (FPR) of 0.13% [17]. The application of cfDNA includes quantitative and qualitative methods. The change of cfDNA's quantity may alert us to tumor gene mutations, diseases' progression, and help prognosis prediction [18]. Elevated concentrations of cfDNA are related to cancer, pregnancy, autoimmune disease, or myocardial infarction [18]. The abnormal cffDNA quantity reflects neonatal hemolytic, preeclampsia (PE), and so on. In prenatal diagnosis, rheumatic heart disease (RhD), sex-related diseases, single-gene disorders, such as β-thalassemia, and cartilage dysplasia are in the diagnosable range [14, 17]. Quantitative analysis methods include spectrophotometer, enzyme-linked immunosorbent assay (ELISA), and real-time fluorescence quantitative PCR (qPCR). Qualitative analysis methods can be used to detect activation or inactivation mutations of *Ras*, *P53*, and other tumor suppressor genes, as well as changes in the DNA immunoglobulin heavy chain [18].

Unfortunately, due to the low concentrations of cfDNA, such determination is only feasible by ultra-accurate devices [19]. Including next-generation sequencing (NGS), most methods are still restricted to targeted genomic loci [20]. Until now, only a few noninvasive attempts have been made.

3.2 Epigenomics

For genomes, not only do sequences contain genetic information, but modifications can also record genetic information. Epigenomics is the field of studying epigenetic modifications at the level of the genome. Epigenetic modifications act on intracellular DNA and its packaging proteins, histones, and are used to regulate genomic function, as manifested by DNA methylation and post-translational modifications of histones, molecular markers that affect the architecture, integrity, and assembly of chromosomes, as well as the ability of DNA to approach its regulatory elements, and chromatin to interact with functional nuclear complexes. Epigenetic biomarkers, including DNA methylation and histone modifications, are increasingly used for disease diagnosis because of their greater specificity and generalizability.

For prenatal diagnosis, epigenomics has a very extensive application. According to recent research, the level of DNA methylation is related to prenatal alcohol exposure (PAE) [21, 22]. Fetal alcohol spectrum disorders (FASD), however, are a consequence of PAE. Alcohol can affect the phenotype of adult mice by modifying the epigenotype of early mouse embryos. Children with FASD may have unique DNA methylation deficiencies, which suggests the further use of biomarkers in the future. In addition, the translation of non-coding RNA, as microRNAs (miRNAs) into proteins, is part of epigenetic regulation. Differential expression of miRNAs is a potential NIPD of fetal coronary artery disease by abnormal pregnancy-associated miRNAs [23].

3.3 Transcriptomics

Transcriptomics is the field that studies gene transcription and transcriptional regulation in cells at the global level. The transcriptome is the total of all RNAs that living cells can transcribe and is an important tool for studying cellular phenotype and function. Transcriptomics is a diagnostic tool based on providing information about the expression of specific genes under specific conditions, which can infer the function of corresponding unknown genes and reveal the mechanism of action of specific regulatory genes. Therefore, transcriptomics is applied to markers in diagnosis. The technology of microarray, serial analysis of gene expression (SAGE), and massively parallel signature sequencing can be applied to the discovery of biomarkers [24].

In terms of application, microarray technology has become one of the leading techniques for prenatal diagnosis in terms of detection rate and accuracy of results [25]. Chromosome microarray analysis (CMA) is applied to the clinical diagnosis of the genetic cause of congenital heart disease (CHD) [26], which is a pioneered new method to improve the detection rate of CHD in children [27]. Biomarkers relevant for the diagnosis of CHD can be applied using multi-omics techniques [28]. This will be described in detail below.

3.4 Proteomics

Proteins are the main carriers of biological functions. Proteomics refers to the study of proteins, including the dynamic changes in protein composition, the analysis of intracellular expression levels and modification states, the understanding of the interactions and connections between proteins, and the elucidation of the rules of protein regulation activity. In conclusion, proteomics mainly involves the study of proteomic expression patterns and functional patterns of protein functional groups. Proteomics determines the basic functional properties of proteins through the identification of their species and structures. Based on the relevant studies of proteins, proteomics has a relevant role in biomarkers.

Proteomics has relevant applications in prenatal diagnosis. In the prenatal diagnosis of biomarkers for trisomy 21, proteomics has been applied in large and multiple ways. Differential protein expression can be identified in the urinary proteome by liquid chromatography–tandem mass spectrometry (LC–MS/MS) analysis to improve the detection of prenatal trisomy 21 [29]. Similarly, mass spectrometry and selective response monitoring (SRM) can be used to screen for differentially expressed proteins in the proteome of maternal serum as biomarkers for trisomy 21.

3.5 Metabonomics

Most of the life activities within a cell occur at the metabolic level, so changes in the metabolites of the cell can more directly reflect the cell's environment. Metabolomics can determine the composition of all small molecules in a cell, map their dynamic patterns of change, create a systematic metabolic map, and determine the link between changes and biological processes. Metabolomics focuses on biological fluids as the object of study, mainly urine and blood. Because of the abundance of endogenous products in blood and the noninvasive nature of urine collection, these body fluids are widely utilized. Compared with genomics and proteomics, metabolomics is more closely related to clinical practice [30]. Based on this advantage, research related to biomarkers is closely affiliated with the application of metabolomics [30].

Non-targeted metabolomics is a powerful tool that can provide a new approach to prenatal diagnosis [31]. It can be utilized for the discovery of affected metabolic pathways and therefore helps to propose potential biomarkers. The search for prenatal biomarkers in preterm birth (PTB) has made full use of metabolomic approaches. Predictive biomarkers of PTB were identified by analysis of prenatal maternal body fluids (amniotic fluid, maternal urine/maternal blood, and cervicovaginal fluid) using nuclear magnetic resonance spectroscopy or mass spectrometry-based methods [32].

4. Application of biomarkers for prenatal diagnosis

4.1 Disorder of pregnancy

4.1.1 Preeclampsia (PE)

PE is a pregnancy-specific syndrome, affecting 3–5% of pregnant women. It is characterized by edemas, proteinuria, and high blood pressure. In women with PE dysfunction of many organs, including liver and kidney, fetus growth restriction is also observed. If untreated, PE may lead to death. In some low-income countries, PE is one of the main causes of maternal and child mortality [33–35].

Hsu et al. identified differentially expressed proteins in serum samples obtained from pregnant women with severe PE and control participants through two-dimensional gel electrophoresis (2-DE) [36]. Then additional serum samples were analyzed by immunoassay for validation. Ten protein spots were discovered to be upregulated in women with PE. Serum α1-antitrypsin, α1-microglobulin, and clusterin levels of

PE patients were significantly higher compared to those in the normal participants [36]. Blankley et al. used isobaric tagging to identify certain potential biomarker proteins in plasma obtained at 15 weeks gestation from nulliparous women who later developed PE. The results confirmed the high accuracy of the pregnancy-specific beta-1-glycoprotein 9 (PSG9) as a potential biomarker for the prenatal diagnosis of PE [37]. Kolialexi et al. collected blood samples from pregnant women at 11–13 weeks of gestation and these women were followed up until delivery. Compared to controls, twelve proteins were differentially expressed in the plasma of women who subsequently developed PE [38, 39].

A systematic review had examined 13 studies, 11 of 13 had found an increase in cfDNA among women who subsequently developed PE [39, 40]. Moreover, four studies examining early-onset or severe PE found increased cfDNA levels compared to disease onset [37]. In one study, the median levels and multiples of the median (MoM) values of *HYP2*, a cfDNA marker, were significantly higher in the preeclampsia and hypertensive disorders of pregnancy groups at 6–14 and 15–23 weeks' gestation compared with controls [39, 41]. *HYP2*, located on chromosome 13, is hypermethylated in the placenta and maternal blood cells. *HYP2* has been studied as an epigenetic marker for total cfDNA [42].

4.1.2 Intrauterine growth restriction (IUGR)

Intrauterine growth restriction (i.e., fetal growth restriction) refers to poor growth of the fetus in the uterus during pregnancy. IUGR is defined by evidence of reduced growth and clinical features of malnutrition [43]. IUGR could cause a baby to be small for gestational age (SGA), which is often defined as a weight below the 10th percentile for gestational age, resulting in low birth weight at the end of pregnancy [36].

Current methods of detection commonly include the measurement of symphysis fundal height (SFH) [44], ultrasound biometry, and doppler ultrasonography. Recently, most interest has been put in novel approaches to screening, including the testing of maternal serum biomarkers and nucleic acids, proteins, vesicles, and metabolites [45].

One study showed that pro-angiogenic placenta growth factor (PlGF) and soluble fms-like tyrosine kinase-1 (sFlt-1) in the first trimester could increase the sensitivity of detection for early-onset IUGR to 86% and 66% for late-onset IUGR through a larger cohort of 9150 women [46]. Based on a multi-parametric method in the third trimester, Miranda et al. designed a nested case–control cohort study in 1590 pregnant women. Their integrated model contained maternal risk factors, estimated fetal weight (EFW), PlGF, unconjugated estriol, and Uterine artery (Ut) Doppler, achieving a sensitivity of 61% for SGA increasing to 77% for IUGR [47]. In addition, it was also proven that low PlGF (< 5th centile) could indicate IUGR with underlying placental pathology with a specificity of 75% and sensitivity of 98% [48].

Like cfDNA, circulating placental RNA (cpRNA) can also be detected in blood, plasma, serum urine, and amniotic fluid in the first trimester [49, 50]. It has been indicated that compared to those who deliver infants in the normal birth weight range, serum cpRNA, cord blood metabolites, urinary metabolites, and amino acid levels in women who develop IUGR would be changed. Future techniques for the detection of specific analytes may focus on microarrays, digital polymerase chain reaction, and NGS, which could identify some RNA analogs. These novel types of more sophisticated biomarkers are the potential to distinguish certain types of IUGR. However, since placental contributions are more common, chances are that such biomarkers would have to outperform PlGF. This kind of method is increasingly becoming a more effective screening and diagnostic tool in the diagnosis of IUGR.

4.2 Genetic disorders

4.2.1 Down syndrome

The most common chromosomal disorder is trisomy 21 [51], also known as Down syndrome, with an incidence of 1 per 800 live births [52]. Common biomarkers used for diagnosing Down syndrome include pregnancy-associated plasma protein-A (PAPP-A), β-human chorionic gonadotropin (β-hCG), alpha-fetoprotein (AFP), Estriol (uE3), dimeric inhibin-A (DIA), etc. [52, 53]. These protein measurements are combined with age, race, weight, number of fetuses in the current gestation, diabetes status, and gestational age to provide a risk estimate. For example, PAPP-A and β-hCG levels are higher in Southeast Asian women compared to Caucasian women, and the serum marker levels in twin pregnancies are approximately twice those found in singleton pregnancies [54].

Usually decreased level of PAPP-A is an indicator for Down syndrome and trisomy 18, whereas the increased level of β-hCG suggests a risk of Down syndrome. These are the two most used serum biomarkers for Down syndrome detection and maternal serum screening (MSS) is often performed with nuchal translucency ultrasound screening. The integration of the two methods is known as enhanced first-trimester screening (eFTs). In most cases ultrasound screening can be diagnostic, MSS is intended only to identify women with pregnancies at increased risk [52]. Further diagnostic methods include cell-free fetal DNA screening (cfDNA screening), amniocentesis, CVS, etc. [55].

One thing has to be noticed during the prenatal screening. In the cases of the vanishing-twin syndrome, the PAPP-A level could be affected by the demise of the twin, and thus should not be used as a means of diagnosis except with alternative adjustments [56]. MSS and eFTs can also be done for the detection of other aneuploidies [57], which means aneuploidies can be diagnosed simultaneously.

4.2.2 β-Thalassemia

β-thalassemia is a blood disorder that reduces the production of hemoglobin. Although studies concerned have suggested that several cord blood serum markers have potential diagnostic value, they have not been worked in application [58]. The relatively mature enough technique is the GthapScreen HBB kit, which involves several STR markers. The DNA samples are purified from blood, amniotic fluid, and CVS. Advantages of this technique include perfect accuracy and no need to consider multiple pregnancies [59].

4.2.3 Gaucher disease (GD)

GD is an autosomal recessive lysosomal storage disorder arising predominantly from mutations in the gene *GBA1* [60], which encodes β-glucocerebrosidase. Insufficient amounts of the hydrolase result in glucosyl sphingosine (GluSph) accumulating in the reticuloendothelial cells of the liver, spleen, bone, and lung, as well as the brain in the rarer disease subtypes. Biomarkers applied in prenatal diagnosis include glucocerebrosidase, which is from cultured amniocytes or chorionic villi cells. However molecular analysis of pathogenic GD mutation is still the preferred method of choice in the prenatal diagnosis of Gaucher disease [61].

DOI: http://dx.doi.org/10.5772/intechopen.104981

4.2.4 Other aneuploidies

Trisomy 18 and trisomy 13 are the second and third most common autosomal trisomy, respectively, with the incidence being 1 in 7500 and 1 in 15,000 live births [52, 62]. Fetuses with trisomy 18 and 13 often experience intrauterine fetal demise [63, 64]. In the late first trimester, average levels of PAPP-A and free β-hCG tend to be lower in pregnancies with trisomy 18 compared with unaffected pregnancies [63]. However, it is shown in related research that ultrasound findings in the first and second trimester for trisomy 18 seem to be more effective than biochemical screening, thus the combination of sonography, triple test, and amniocentesis makes sense [65]. As for trisomy 13, a decrease in maternal serum-free β-hCG and PAPP-A and an increase in fetal nuchal translucency always come into existence. However, the use of biochemical markers in maternal serum as a screening tool for trisomy 13 seems to be less promising than for other aneuploidies, such as trisomy 21 and trisomy 18 [64]. By using different markers, the hap screen kit technique mentioned in the β-thalassemia part could also be applied in the diagnosis of disorders of chromosomes 21, 18, 13, X, and Y [59].

4.3 Congenital structural malformations

4.3.1 Neural tube defects (NTDs)

NTDs are serious congenital malformation disorders. The neural tube is the central nervous system of the fetus. On the 15th to 17th day of the embryo, the nervous system begins to develop, and by about the 22nd day of the embryo, the two sides of the neural fold begin to close to each other, forming a canal called the neural tube. The embryo closes the anterior foramen and posterior phase on the 24th, 25th, and 26th day. The central neural tube is the part of the embryo that develops into the brain, spinal cord, back of the head, and spine. If the central nervous canal does not develop properly, the above-mentioned parts may be defective when the baby is born. The main manifestations of fetal neural tube malformations are anencephaly, cerebral bulge, cerebrospinal meningeal bulge, and spina bifida [66].

The first biomarker for prenatal testing is related to neural tube defect screening AFP [67]. Maternal serum AFP levels are closely related to the developmental status of the neural tube. Serum AFP screening is generally performed between 15 and 21 weeks of pregnancy. Blood samples can be collected in the form of liquid, whole blood, or dried blood. Studies have shown that anencephalic children have AFP levels that are 6.4 the normal gestation-specific median. In cases associated with spina bifida, AFP levels were 3.8 the normal gestation-specific median. As technology continues to develop and advance, the accuracy of screening for AFP as a biomarker for NTDs has increased and the detection rate of false positives has further decreased.

Recent studies have explored new biomarkers to detect NTDs. AFP-associated maternal serum α-fetoprotein variants L2 and L3 (AFP-L2 and AFP-L3) are more accurate predictors of fetal open neural tube defects (ONTD) with high sensitivity and specificity [68]. In addition, amniotic fluid glial fibrillary acidic protein (AF-GFAP) was shown to be a valid diagnostic biomarker for NTDs by proteomic studies [69]. NTDs were positive in the open stage and negative in the closed stage when the threshold was above 0.2 ng/mL. This confirms that amniotic glial fibrillary acidic protein is a biomarker for the diagnosis of open NTDs and has a negative predictive role in the detection of closed NTDs.

In noninvasive prenatal screening, in addition to conventional methods for AFP level changes, a breakthrough was made in biomarkers of NTDs using isobaric tags for relative and absolute quantitation (iTRAQ) quantitative proteomics technology [70]. The expression of proprotein convertase subtilisin/kexin type 9 (PCSK9) differed in rat fetuses at different developmental stages [71], with a significant decrease in NTD pregnancy serum and a progressive increase in normal pregnancy and embryonic development serum. Although the possibility of using biomarkers for prenatal testing in humans has not been confirmed, it has a promising prospect.

4.3.2 Congenital heart disease (CHD)

CHD is the most pervasive type of congenital malformation, making up for approximately 28% of congenital malformations. Refers to anatomical abnormalities resulting from abnormal formation or development of the heart and great blood vessels during embryonic development. The heart and great vessels are abnormal at birth, including right-to-right shunt, right-to-left shunt, and no shunt. Tetralogy of Fallot is the most common type of left-to-right shunt CHD [72].

In terms of invasive prenatal testing, the search for suitable biomarkers for prenatal testing is broadly based on two routes—cord blood and amniotic fluid. In the amniotic fluid of fetuses with CHD [73], uric acid and proline were found to be significantly elevated by metabolomic analysis. Among them, uric acid has good specificity and sensitivity and has a promising potential to become a biomarker. Cord blood can be used as a prenatal biological marker for a variety of diseases, including CHD [74]. Analysis of miRNAs reveals significantly elevated expression of miRNA-1, miRNA-208, and miRNA-499, which have the prospect to be biomarkers for CHD.

Noninvasive prenatal testing for CHD is more common. The techniques of proteomics have been used more often in the diagnosis of CHD [75]. In maternal serum [76], proteomic analysis is used to find peptides specifically expressed in fetuses with tetralogy of Fallot. In addition to peptides, it has been shown that maternal serum concentrations of tumor necrosis factor-alpha, vascular endothelial growth factor-d, and heparin-binding epidermal growth factor-like growth factor are associated with CHD with a high degree of specificity [77].

4.3.3 Cleft lip and palate (CLP)

CLP is the most pervasive congenital malformation in the oral and maxillofacial region, mainly due to certain pathogenic factors that cause fetal facial development disorders between the fourth and tenth week of pregnancy [78]. Genetics and maternal conditions are the main causes of CLP. Prenatal diagnosis of fetal CLP is mainly carried out by fetal ultrasound images [78]. However, this technique has many limitations; maternal weight and fetal position can interfere with the diagnostic results. Prenatal diagnosis of CLP is prone to misdiagnosis and underdiagnosis [78].

The discovery of prenatal biomarkers for CLP has made it possible to improve the accuracy of prenatal diagnosis [78, 79]. Three pregnancy-associated PIWI-interacting RNAs (piRNAs) biomarkers (hsa-pri-009228, hsa-pri-016659, and hsa-pri-020496) are reported able to distinguish CLP fetuses from normal fetuses. In CLP fetuses, the expression of piRNAs biomarkers was down-regulated with high accuracy, which is of high clinical value. CLP was first discovered as a related prenatal biomarker, which has high clinical value as a non-invasive detection method.

4.3.4 Congenital glaucoma

Congenital glaucoma is a congenital abnormality of the atrial angle structure due to developmental disorders during embryonic life, which blocks the channels for atrial fluid drainage, resulting in increased intraocular pressure and increasing the size of the entire eye. Glaucoma is a disease that causes damage to the optic nerve. When the intraocular pressure increases, it can lead to damage to the optic nerve fibers and cause visual field defects.

The discovery of biomarkers associated with congenital glaucoma offers the possibility of prenatal diagnosis. Human fetuses with cytochrome p4501B1 mutations are more likely to have congenital glaucoma [80]. Detection of cytochrome p4501B1 expression reveals that fetuses with congenital glaucoma have delayed ocular tissue development and decreased cytochrome p4501B1 protein expression, thus increasing oxidative stress biomarkers.

4.3.5 Achondroplasia

Chondrodysplasia is an autosomal dominant disorder with a point mutation in the short arm of chromosome 4, a congenital developmental abnormality due to a defect in endochondral ossification, mainly affecting long bones. A large proportion of cases of chondrodysplasia are stillborn or die in the neonatal period.

The diagnosis of chondrodysplasia is largely dependent on breakthroughs in noninvasive prenatal diagnostic methods. Analysis of cellular free DNA using PCR and restriction endonuclease digestion (PCR-red) is the dominant method for noninvasive prenatal detection of monogenic diseases including chondrodysplasia [81]. A novel NGS assay was found to be more sensitive and specific for chondrodysplasia. In addition, cffDNA may be a useful biomarker for NIPD. Related studies have confirmed the significance of the detection of *FGFR3* gene mutations in cffDNA for the diagnosis of early maternal chondrodysplasia. Based on this biomarker, a novel DNA sensor for detecting disease-causing mutant genes was designed, which is very sensitive for genetic detection in poor cartilage [82].

5. Conclusion

Biomarkers based on multi-omics have a wide variety of applications in prenatal diagnosis, and samples are collected either through invasive or noninvasive ways. Maternal serum biomarkers are ideal diagnostic indexes because of their convenience and security. However, in the present stage, invasive techniques, such as amniocentesis and CVS, are often required to confirm the preliminary result, although they carry a risk of miscarriage and need people with specialty to operate them. Researches on noninvasive techniques are now on the rise. Despite the high cost, noninvasive techniques, such as cfDNA, are quite risk-free and accurate, which is promising for the future.

Author details

Tong Wang[1,2,3], Jiahe Xu[1,2,4], Lin Wang[1,2,4], Xiumin Cui[1,2,4], Yan Yan[5], Qiuqin Tang[6*] and Wei Wu[1,2*]

1 State Key Laboratory of Reproductive Medicine, Institute of Toxicology, Nanjing Medical University, Nanjing, China

2 Key Laboratory of Modern Toxicology of Ministry of Education, School of Public Health, Nanjing Medical University, Nanjing, China

3 The Stomatological College of Nanjing Medical University, Nanjing, China

4 The First Clinical Medical College, Nanjing Medical University, Nanjing, China

5 Nanjing Hanwei Public Health Research Institute, Nanjing, China

6 Department of Obstetrics, Women's Hospital of Nanjing Medical University, Nanjing Maternity and Child Health Care Hospital, Nanjing, China

*Address all correspondence to: t19871004@sina.com and wwu@njmu.edu.cn

References

[1] Chen LZ, Zhang M, Ma W, et al. The main advances in the application of proteomics in prenatal diagnosis. Chinese Journal of General Practice. 2018;**16**(3):461-464

[2] Palomaki GE, Kloza EM, Lambert-Messerlian GM, et al. DNA sequencing of maternal plasma to detect down syndrome: An international clinical validation study. Genetics in Medicine. 2011;**13**(11):913-920

[3] Herzenberg LA, Bianchi DW, Schroder J, Cann HM, Iverson GM. Fetal cells in the blood of pregnant women: Detection and enrichment by fluorescence-activated cell sorting. Proceedings of the National Academy of Sciences. 1979;**76**(3):1453-1455

[4] Benn P, Borrell A, Cuckle H, et al. Prenatal detection of down syndrome using massively parallel sequencing (MPS): A rapid response statement from a committee on behalf of the Board of the International Society for prenatal diagnosis, 24 October 2011: A rapid response statement from a committee on behalf of the board of the ISPD, 24 October 2011. Prenatal Diagnosis. 2012;**32**(1):1-2

[5] Fan HC, Blumenfeld YJ, Chitkara U, Hudgins L, Quake SR. Noninvasive diagnosis of fetal aneuploidy by shotgun sequencing DNA from maternal blood. Proceedings of the National Academy of Sciences. 2008;**105**(42):16266-16271

[6] Yurkiewicz IR, Korf BR, Lehmann LS. Prenatal whole-genome sequencing — Is the quest to know a Fetus's future ethical? The New England Journal of Medicine. 2014;**370**(3):195-197

[7] Imudia AN, Kumar S, Diamond MP, DeCherney AH, Armant DR. Transcervical retrieval of fetal cells in the practice of modern medicine: A review of the current literature and future direction. Fertility and Sterility. 2010;**93**(6):1725-1730

[8] Kabra M. Prenatal diagnosis. Indian Journal of Pediatric. 2003;**70**(1):81-85

[9] Gur O, Chang CL, Jain R, et al. High-purity isolation of rare single cells from blood using a tiered microchip system. PLoS One. 2020;**15**(3):e0229949

[10] Szilágyi M, Pös O, Márton É, et al. Circulating cell-free nucleic acids: Main characteristics and clinical application. International Journal of Molecular Science. 2020;**21**(18):6827

[11] Rabinowitz T, Polsky A, Golan D, et al. Bayesian-based noninvasive prenatal diagnosis of single-gene disorders. Genome Research. 2019;**29**(3):428-438

[12] Mandel P, Metais P. Nuclear acids in human blood plasma. Comptes Rendus Des Séances De La Société De Biologie Et De Ses Filiales. 1948;**142**(3-4):241-243

[13] Leon SA, Green A, Yaros MJ, Shapiro B. Radioimmunoassay for nanogram quantities of DNA. Journal of Immunological Methods. 1975;**9**(2):157-164

[14] Lo YMD, Corbetta N, Chamberlain PF, et al. Presence of fetal DNA in maternal plasma and serum. Lancet. 1997;**350**(9076):485-487

[15] Snyder MW, Kircher M, Hill AJ, Daza RM, Shendure J. Cell-free DNA comprises an In vivo nucleosome footprint that informs its tissues-of-origin. Cell. 2016;**164**(1-2):57-68

[16] Al Nakib M, Desbrière R, Bonello N. Total and fetal cell-free DNA analysis in maternal blood as markers of placental insufficiency in intrauterine growth restriction. Fetal Diagnosis & Therapy. 2009;**26**(1):24-28

[17] Gil MM, Accurti V, Santacruz B, Plana MN, Nicolaides KH. Analysis of cell-free DNA in maternal blood in screening for aneuploidies: Updated meta-analysis. Ultrasound in Obstetrics & Gynecology. 2017;**50**(3):302-314

[18] Duan Y, Zhang H, Yu S, et al. Advances in the medical research and clinical applications on the plasma DNA. Translational Pediatrics. 2014;**3**(2):140-148

[19] Lun FM, Tsui NB, Chan KC, et al. Noninvasive prenatal diagnosis of monogenic diseases by digital size selection and relative mutation dosage on DNA in maternal plasma. Proceedings of the National Academy of Sciences of the United States of America. 2008;**105**(50):19920-19925

[20] Lam KW, Jiang P, Liao GJ, et al. Noninvasive prenatal diagnosis of monogenic diseases by targeted massively parallel sequencing of maternal plasma: Application to beta-thalassemia. Clinical Chemistry. 2012;**58**(10):1467-1475

[21] Kaminen-Ahola N. Fetal alcohol spectrum disorders: Genetic and epigenetic mechanisms. Prenatal Diagnosis. 2020;**40**(9):1185-1192

[22] Ke Z, Liu Y, Wang X, et al. Cyanidin-3-glucoside ameliorates ethanol neurotoxicity in the developing brain. Journal of Neuroscience Research. 2011;**89**(10):1676-1684

[23] Gai W, Sun K. Epigenetic biomarkers in cell-free DNA and applications in liquid biopsy. Genes (Basel). 2019;**10**(1):32

[24] So AP, Turner RF, Haynes CA. Minimizing loss of sequence information in SAGE Ditags by modulating the temperature dependent 3′ --> 5′ exonuclease activity of DNA polymerases on 3′-terminal Isoheptyl amino groups. Biotechnology and Bioengineering. 2006;**94**(1):54-65

[25] Suela J, López-Expósito I, Querejeta ME, et al. Recommendations for the use of microarrays in prenatal diagnosis. Medicina Clínica. 2017;**148**(7):328.e1-328.e8

[26] Gupta D, Mowitz ME, Lopez-Colon D, Nixon CS, Vyas HV, Co-Vu JG. Effect of prenatal diagnosis on hospital costs in complete transposition of the great arteries. Prenatal Diagnosis. 2018;**38**(8):567-571

[27] Wu X-L, Li R, Fu F, et al. Chromosome microarray analysis in the investigation of children with congenital heart disease. BMC Pediatrics. 2017;**17**(1):117

[28] Chen L, Guan J, Wei Q, Yuan Z, Zhang M. Potential role of "omics" technique in prenatal diagnosis of congenital heart defects. Clinica Chimica Acta. 2018;**482**:185-190

[29] Gao L, Zhang J, Ran X, et al. Urinary proteomics for noninvasive prenatal screening of trisomy 21: New biomarker candidates. OMICS. 2021;**25**(11):738-744

[30] Shahid M, Yeon A, Kim J. Metabolomic and Lipidomic approaches to identify biomarkers for bladder cancer and interstitial cystitis (review). Molecular Medicine Reports. 2020;**22**(6):5003-5011

[31] Parfieniuk E, Zbucka-Kretowska M, Ciborowski M, Kretowski A, Barbas C.

Untargeted metabolomics: An overview of its usefulness and future potential in prenatal diagnosis. Expert Review of Proteomics. 2018;**15**(10):809-816

[32] Gil AM, Duarte D. Biofluid metabolomics in preterm birth research. Reproductive Science. 2018;**25**(7):967-977

[33] Alfirevic Z, Navaratnam K, Mujezinovic F. Amniocentesis and chorionic villus sampling for prenatal diagnosis. Cochrane Database of Systematic Reviews. 2017;**9**(9):1-174

[34] Filipek A, Jurewicz E. Preeclampsia - a disease of pregnant women. Postepy Biochemii. 2018;**64**(4):232-229

[35] Mol BWJ, Roberts CT, Thangaratinam S, Magee LA, de Groot CJM, Hofmeyr GJ. Pre-eclampsia. Lancet. 2016;**387**(10022):999-1011

[36] Hsu TY, Hsieh TT, Yang KD, et al. Proteomic profiling reveals α1-antitrypsin, α1-microglobulin, and clusterin as preeclampsia-related serum proteins in pregnant women. Taiwanese Journal of Obstetrics & Gynecology. 2015;**54**(5):499-504

[37] Blankley RT, Fisher C, Westwood M, et al. A label-free selected reaction monitoring workflow identifies a subset of pregnancy specific glycoproteins as potential predictive markers of early-onset pre-eclampsia. Molecular & Cellular Proteomics. 2013;**12**(11):3148-3159

[38] Kolialexi A, Tsangaris GT, Sifakis S, et al. Plasma biomarkers for the identification of women at risk for early-onset preeclampsia. Expert Review of Proteomics. 2017;**14**(3):269-276

[39] Kwak DW, Kim SY, Kim HJ, Lim JH, Kim YH, Ryu HM. Maternal Total cell-free DNA in preeclampsia with and without intrauterine growth restriction. Scientific Reports. 2020;**10**(1):11848

[40] McCarthy FP, Ryan RM, Chappell LC. Prospective biomarkers in preterm preeclampsia: A review. Pregnancy Hypertension. 2018;**14**:72-78

[41] Kim SY, Kim HJ, Park SY, Han YJ, Choi JS, Ryu HM. Early prediction of hypertensive disorders of pregnancy using cell-free Fetal DNA, cell-free Total DNA, and biochemical markers. Fetal Diagnosis & Therapy. 2016;**40**(4):255-262

[42] Hahn S, Rusterholz C, Hosli I, Lapaire O. Cell-free nucleic acids as potential markers for preeclampsia. Placenta. 2011;**32**(Supplemental 1): S17-S20

[43] Kesavan K, Devaskar SU. Intrauterine growth restriction. Pediatric Clinics of North America. 2019;**66**(2):403-423

[44] Duri K, Gumbo FZ, Munjoma PT, et al. The University of Zimbabwe College of health sciences (UZ-CHS) birth cohort study: Rationale, design and methods. BMC Infectious Diseases. 2020;**20**(1):725

[45] Audette MC, Kingdom JC. Screening for fetal growth restriction and placental insufficiency. Seminars in Fetal and Neonatal Medicine. 2018;**23**(2):119-125

[46] Crovetto F, Triunfo S, Crispi F, et al. First-trimester screening with specific algorithms for early-and late-onset fetal growth restriction. Ultrasound in Obstetrics & Gynecology. 2016;**48**(3):340-348

[47] Miranda J, Rodriguez-Lopez M, Triunfo S, et al. Prediction of fetal growth restriction using estimated

fetal weight vs a combined screening model in the third trimester. Ultrasound in Obstetrics & Gynecology. 2017;**50**:603-611

[48] Benton SJ, McCowan LM, Heazell AEP, et al. Placental growth factor as a marker of fetal growth restriction caused by placental dysfunction. Placenta. 2016;**42**:1-8

[49] Cox B, Leavey K, Nosi U, Wong F, Kingdom J. Placental transcriptome in development and pathology: Expression, function, and methods of analysis. American Journal of Obstetrics and Gynecology. 2015;**213**:S138-S151

[50] Tsui NBY, Jiang P, Wong YF, et al. Maternal plasma RNA sequencing for genome-wide transcriptomic profiling and identification of pregnancy associated transcripts. Clinical Chemistry. 2014;**60**:954-962

[51] Perry JC, Pakkenberg B, Vann SD. Striking reduction in neurons and glial cells in anterior thalamic nuclei of older patients with down syndrome. Neurobiology of Aging. 2019;**75**:54-61

[52] Carlson LM, Vora NL. Prenatal diagnosis: Screening and diagnostic tools. Obstetrics and Gynecology Clinics of North America. 2017;**44**(2):245-256

[53] Chaveeva P, Wright A, Syngelaki A, et al. Second trimester serum biomarker screen for Fetal aneuploidies as a predictor of preterm delivery: A population-based study. Gynecologic and Obstetric Investigation. 2019;**84**(4):326-333

[54] Rink BD, Norton ME. Screening for fetal aneuploidy. Seminars in Perinatology. 2016;**40**(1):35-43

[55] Huang T, Gibbons C, Rashid S, et al. Prenatal screening for trisomy 21: A comparative performance and cost analysis of different screening strategies. BMC Pregnancy and Childbirth. 2020;**20**(1):713

[56] Chaveeva P, Wright A, Syngelaki A, et al. First-trimester screening for trisomies in pregnancies with vanishing twin. Ultrasound in Obstetrics & Gynecology. 2020;**55**(3):326-331

[57] Wang Y, Li S, Wang W, et al. Cell-free DNA screening for sex chromosome aneuploidies by non-invasive prenatal testing in maternal plasma. Molecular Cytogenetics. 2020;**12**(13):10

[58] Zhan W, Guo H, Hu S, et al. Comparison of cord blood hematological parameters among normal, α-thalassemia, and β-thalassemia fetuses between 17 and 38 weeks of gestation. Scientific Reports. 2021;**11**(1):3844

[59] Sharifi Z, Rahiminejad F, Joudaki A, et al. Development and validation of a novel panel of 16 STR markers for simultaneous diagnosis of β-thalassemia, aneuploidy screening, maternal cell contamination detection and fetal sample authenticity in PND and PGD/PGS cases. Scientific Reports. 2019;**9**(1):7452

[60] Vilageliu L, Grinberg D. Involvement of Gaucher disease mutations in Parkinson disease. Current Protein & Peptide Science. 2017;**18**(7):758-764

[61] Bodamer OA, Hung C. Laboratory and genetic evaluation of Gaucher disease. Wiener Medizinische Wochenschrift (1946). 2010;**160**(23-24): 600-604

[62] Goel N, Morris JK, Tucker D, et al. Trisomy 13 and 18-prevalence and mortality-a multi-registry population-based analysis. American Journal of Medical Genetics. 2019;**179**(12):2382-2392

[63] Bestwick JP, Huttly WJ, Wald NJ. Serum marker truncation limits in first trimester antenatal screening for trisomy 18. Journal of Medical Screening. 2018;**25**(4):169-173

[64] Rajs B, Pasternok M, Nocuń A, et al. Clinical article: Screening for trisomy 13 using traditional combined screening versus an ultrasound-based protocol. The Journal of Maternal-Fetal & Neonatal Medicine. 2021;**34**(7):1048-1054

[65] Niknejadi M, Ahmadi F, Akhbari F, Afsharian P. Sonographic findings in partial type of trisomy 18. International Journal of Fertility & Sterility. 2014;7(4):349-352

[66] Greene NDE, Copp AJ. Neural tube defects. Annual Review of Neuroscience. 2014;**37**:221-242

[67] Cuckle H, Maymon R. Development of prenatal screening--a historical overview. Seminars in Perinatology. 2016;**40**(1):12-22

[68] Chen Y, Wang X, Lu S, Huang J, Zhang L, Hu W. The diagnostic accuracy of maternal serum alpha-fetoprotein variants (AFP-L2 and AFP-L3) in predicting fetal open neural tube defects and abdominal wall defects. Clinica Chimica Acta. 2020;**507**:125-131

[69] Lopez J, Mikaelian I, Gonzalo P. Amniotic fluid glial fibrillary acidic protein (AF-GFAP), a biomarker of open neural tube defects. Prenatal Diagnosis. 2013;**33**(10):990-995

[70] An D, Wei X, Li H, et al. Identification of PCSK9 as a novel serum biomarker for the prenatal diagnosis of neural tube defects using iTRAQ quantitative proteomics. Scientific Reports. 2015;**5**:17559

[71] Wang C, Zheng Q, Zhang M, Lu H. Lack of ethnic differences in the pharmacokinetics and pharmacodynamics of evolocumab between Caucasian and Asian populations. British Journal of Clinical Pharmacology. 2019;**85**(1):114-125

[72] Helbing WA, Roest AA, Niezen RA, et al. ECG predictors of ventricular arrhythmias and biventricular size and wall mass in tetralogy of Fallot with pulmonary regurgitation. Heart. 2002;**88**(5):515-519

[73] Li Y, Sun Y, Yang L, et al. Analysis of biomarkers for congenital heart disease based on maternal amniotic fluid metabolomics. Frontiers in Cardiovascular Medicine. 2021;**8**:671191

[74] Kong D, Li H, Ren C, Yang W, Zhang Z. MicroRNAs in Fetal umbilical cord blood as a prenatal screening tool for congenital heart disease. Annals of Clinical and Laboratory Science. 2021;**51**(5):705-712

[75] Chen L, Gu H, Li J, et al. Comprehensive maternal serum proteomics identifies the cytoskeletal proteins as non-invasive biomarkers in prenatal diagnosis of congenital heart defects. Scientific Reports. 2016;**6**:19248

[76] Zhuang B, Hu Y, Fan X, et al. Peptidomic analysis of maternal serum to identify biomarker candidates for prenatal diagnosis of tetralogy of Fallot. Journal of Cellular Biochemistry. 2018;**119**(1):468-477

[77] Miyoshi T, Hosoda H, Nakai M, et al. Maternal biomarkers for fetal heart failure in fetuses with congenital heart defects or arrhythmias. American Journal of Obstetrics and Gynecology. 2019;**220**(1):104

[78] Escalon J, Huissoud C, Bisch C, Gonnaud F, Fichez A, Rudigoz RC. Parental impact of 3D/4D ultrasonography

in Fetal cleft lip and palate. Gynecologie Obstetrique Fertilite and Senologie. 2010;**38**(2):101-104

[79] Jia S, Zhang Q, Wang Y, et al. PIWI-interacting RNA sequencing profiles in maternal plasma-derived exosomes reveal novel non-invasive prenatal biomarkers for the early diagnosis of nonsyndromic cleft lip and palate. eBioMedicine. 2021;**65**:103253

[80] Rezaei
Kanavi M, Yazdani S, Elahi E, et al. Prenatal diagnosis of primary congenital glaucoma and histopathological features in a fetal globe with mutations. European Journal of Ophthalmology. 2021;**3**:11206721211051235

[81] Chitty LS, Mason S, Barrett AN, et al. Non-invasive prenatal diagnosis of achondroplasia and thanatophoric dysplasia: Next-generation sequencing allows for a safer, more accurate, and comprehensive approach. Prenatal Diagnosis. 2015;**35**(7):656-662

[82] Chen J, Yu C, Zhao Y, et al. A novel non-invasive detection method for the FGFR3 gene mutation in maternal plasma for a fetal achondroplasia diagnosis based on signal amplification by hemin-MOFs/PtNPs. Biosensors & Bioelectronics. 2017;**91**:892-899

Chapter 10

Prenatal Screening: A Tool to Predict, Prevent, and Prepare

Brinda Sabu and Vidyalekshmy Ranganayaki

Abstract

There has been a considerable reduction in maternal mortality from 6 to 9/1000 live births and infant mortality from 100/1000 live births in the 1900s to less than 0.1/1000 live births and 7/1000 live births, respectively, in the 2000s. This is mostly due to nutritional improvement and obstetric and fetal medicine advancements. However, in the current era, prevention of mortality is not the only goal but also the prevention of morbidity. Thus comes the importance of prenatal screening, which would help us to predict and prevent maternal-fetal complications and in non-preventable conditions to prepare ourselves for optimal care of the mother and fetus. Prenatal screening is thus a test to detect potential health disorders in pregnant mothers or the fetus and to identify a subset who may need additional testing to determine the presence or absence of disease. It is done to categorize mothers into high-risk and low-risk pregnancies to prevent maternal complications, screen the fetus for aneuploidies, anomalies, and growth abnormalities, and decide on any indicated interventions and the time and mode of safe delivery so that an optimal perinatal outcome is achieved. Prenatal screening not only caters to identify fetal complications but also attempts to identify maternal complications early.

Keywords: prenatal screening, aneuploidy, preeclampsia, preterm labor, small for gestational age, fetal anomalies, adverse pregnancy outcomes, preventive strategies, screening models

1. Introduction

In 1929, the Ministry of Health in the UK set forth guidelines advocating for pregnant women to be first seen in the antenatal clinics at 16 weeks, followed by 24 and 28 weeks visits, fortnightly till 36 weeks, and weekly until delivery [1, 2] (**Figure 1a**). However, in 2011, Prof. Nicolaides inverted this pyramid of prenatal care by introducing a new model where a comprehensive assessment of the mother and the fetus is done at 11–13 weeks. According to this "inverted pyramid model", combining the data from maternal characteristics and history along with biophysical and biochemical tests performed on the mother can define the patient-specific risk for a variety of pregnancy complications, namely aneuploidies, preeclampsia, preterm delivery, gestational diabetes, fetal growth restriction, and macrosomia [5]. (**Figure 1b**). In 2017, Ljubic proposed an "extended inverted pyramid of care" based

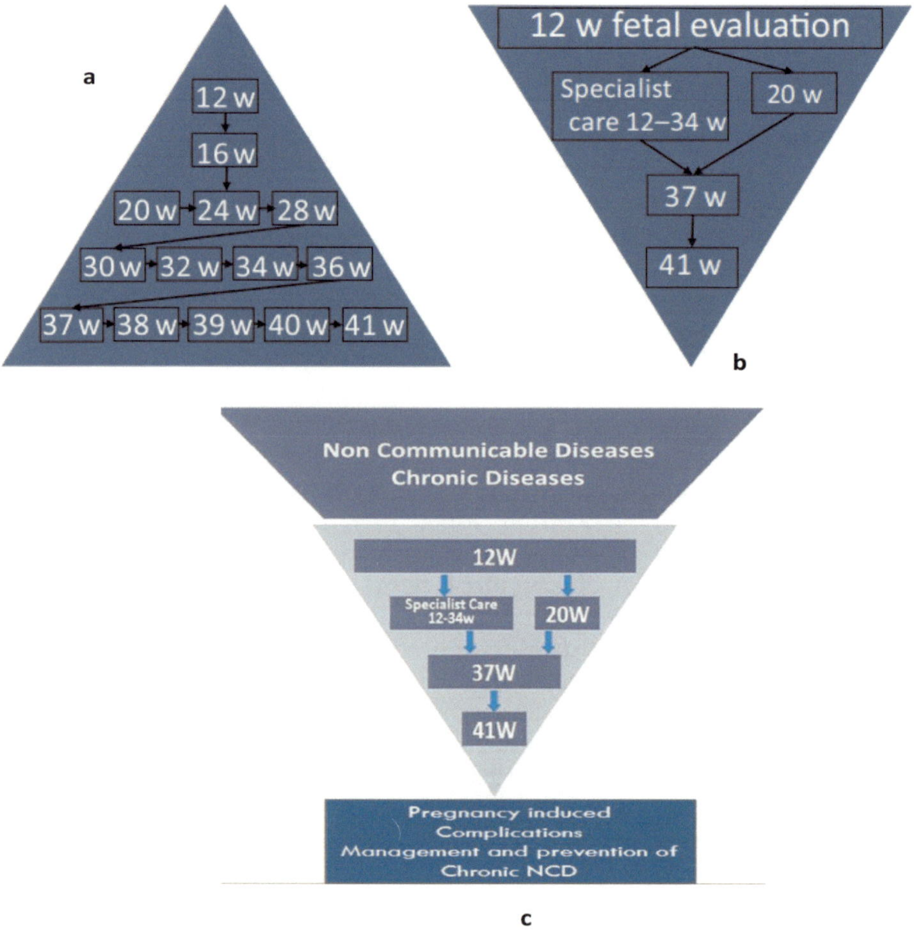

Figure 1.
(a) Pyramid of care in 1929, (b) inverted pyramid of prenatal care (adapted from [3]), (c) three floor model which includes prepregnancy and postpregnancy care (adapted from [4]).

on the concept that the roots of these disorders are dysfunctional placentation and thus must be sought in the earlier period of pregnancy and in the deeper, subcellular level [6]. This means that the changes that lead to insufficient implantation should be sought in the preimplantation period, in the relation between the embryo and endometrium. Prepregnancy approaches such as optimizing maternal comorbidities, adequate weight management, blood pressure and glycemic control, smoking cessation, and spacing pregnancies may improve the placentation leading to an optimal pregnancy outcome [7]. Year 2016 saw the emergence of another model put forward by Moshe and Nicolaides called the "Three-floor model" where the care is extended to prepregnancy and postnatal periods [4] (**Figure 1c**). This model was proposed based on the concept that the health effects of women and their offspring are mediated by epigenetic and genetic pathways contributing to the increased risk of developing noncommunicable diseases (NCD) that are passed onto the next generations, which is a vicious cycle. Thus, this model of care helps in the assessment of NCDs in the prepregnancy period (first floor) and optimizing the disease state followed by the inverted pyramid of care (second floor) starting at 11–14 weeks till delivery, to the postnatal period (third floor) where appropriate management can minimize the long term harmful effects in both mother and her offspring. Hence, this model of prenatal screening, which starts from the prepregnancy period and continues through pregnancy into the postnatal period, would be an ideal screening model, and this would reduce the harmful effects of the epigenetic/genetic factors on the fetus and the mother, thereby reducing the long term development of NCDs.

In this chapter we shall discuss the different screening methods which can be applied to these three floors of prenatal care:

1. First floor—Prepregnancy period

2. Second floor—Inverted pyramid of care from 11 weeks till delivery

3. Third floor—Postnatal period

2. Prepregnancy period

Prepregnancy care aims to identify the women with NCDs and treat them and optimize their disease state. This is done by the family physician or primary obstetrician by gathering patient information either through personal interviews or from electronic records regarding medical, pregnancy, and family history, drug intake, and smoking. A physical examination is done to calculate the BMI and BP and investigations like HbA1C and total cholesterol are conducted. Seven cardiovascular health (CVH) metrics proposed by the American heart association (AHA) are assessed which include four health behaviors (weight, physical activity, smoking, and diet) and three health risk factors (blood pressure, fasting blood glucose, and total cholesterol). Based on these metrics patients are stratified into different risk categories, namely—ideal [8–12], intermediate [4, 7, 13–15], and poor (0–4) categories [13]. Two points are awarded for ideal, one point for intermediate, and zero points for poor, ranging from 0 to 14 [13].

Women who score ideal risk are reassured and advised to plan their families. Those women who score intermediate risk should be referred to either dieticians or physical trainers to optimize their pregnancy issues at hand. The poor score women are referred to a maternal-fetal medicine (MFM) specialist to optimize comorbidities like anemia/hypertension/diabetes, evaluation of the end organs in chronic morbidities, conversion to pregnancy-safe medications, screen for infections, and immunization of varicella/rubella and hepatitis B. Carriers of inherited genetic disorders should be offered counseling and workup by geneticist including index child workup, genetic evaluation for carrier status, and preimplantation genetic diagnosis (PIGD). Periconceptional folic acid should be advised as and where indicated.

3. Inverted pyramid of care

In the 11–14 weeks period, a comprehensive evaluation of the mother is done based on the demographics, medical/obstetric, and family history along with biophysical markers like mean arterial pressure (MAP), biochemical markers like human chorionic gonadotrophin (HCG), pregnancy-associated placental plasma protein A (PAPP-A) and placental growth factor (PLGF), and ultrasound (USG) parameters like nuchal translucency (NT) and uterine artery Doppler pulsatility index (UTPI) thus quantifying the woman's risk for developing any chromosomal aberrations, preeclampsia, spontaneous preterm birth, fetal growth restriction, and gestational diabetes. Thus, they are stratified as low-risk and high-risk pregnancies. Low-risk mothers enter the routine care regimen and high-risk mothers enter the specialist care regimen.

The inverted pyramid of care thus includes:

A. Aneuploidy screening

B. Preeclampsia/SGA screening

C. Screening for preterm labor

D. Screening for diabetes

E. Screening for anomalies

3.1 Aneuploidy screening

Aneuploidy screen has come a long way since its inception in the 1970s. Early detection of Down syndrome is the main objective of prenatal aneuploidy screening since this syndrome is the most common autosomal trisomy among live births which is compatible with life. Trisomy 21 affects 1 per 500 pregnancies with a live birth prevalence of 1 per 740 while trisomy 18 occurs in 1 per 2000 pregnancies and 1 per 6600 live borns, and trisomy 13 is identified in 1 per 5000 pregnancies and 1 per 12,000 live borns [14, 15]. As detection of aneuploidies is also observed in younger age groups, screening is universal in the current era and all pregnant women should be offered screening for aneuploidies. There are two different types of aneuploidy screening:

1. Conventional screening

2. Cell-free DNA-based screening

Conventional screening is the established method of screening using NT performed by USG along with biochemical screening in the first trimester and only biochemical screening in the second trimester. It is further divided into three types:

A. First trimester combined screening

B. Second trimester biochemical screening

C. Combinations of first and second trimester screening: integrated and sequential screens

Cell-free DNA screening which was implemented in 2011, identifies circulating DNA fragments that are primarily placental in origin, from apoptotic trophoblasts [8, 9] and is considered to be the best available screening test with a good positive predictive value, and a very low false positive rate especially when applied appropriately.

3.1.1 Conventional screening

3.1.1.1 First trimester combined screening (FTS)

Components of FTS are as follows:

a. Pretest counseling

b. USG evaluation

c. Biochemical screening/Risk assessment

d. Posttest counseling

3.1.1.1.1 Pretest counseling

Every pregnant woman is counseled regarding the options of undergoing a screening test, diagnostic test, or no test at all, their detection rates and it is completely her choice to proceed with any testing. She is counseled that the purpose of the screening test is to provide information and if the test results come positive, it does not mean that the fetus is affected (false positive) and there is the option of diagnostic testing to confirm the same. Decisions cannot solely be taken based on screening tests. Similarly, it does not mean the fetus is unaffected if the test results come negative (false negative). The benefits of diagnosis, early intervention if affected and the costs of the screening and diagnostic tests are also explained. Additional evaluation and counseling are suggested if a patient has had a previous fetus or neonate with autosomal trisomy, Robertsonian translocation, or other chromosomal abnormality.

3.1.1.1.2 USG evaluation

There has been a paradigm shift in utilizing USG for the detection of aneuploidy markers to early identification of structural and genetic abnormalities. The salient applications of USG in the first trimester are:

i. To calculate the GA

ii. To identify multiple gestations and their chorionicity

iii. To identify aneuploidy markers

iv. To identify major structural malformations

3.1.1.1.2.1 Calculation of GA

Dating is of paramount importance before aneuploidy testing because each screening test is valid only within a specific gestational age window, 11–14 weeks for first trimester screening and 15–21 weeks for second trimester screening. Moreover, when risk assessment is done each component of a screening test should be adjusted for gestational age when calculating multiples of the median, and false positive rates are reduced when gestational age is assessed by USG [10]. Crown-rump length (CRL) is the length of the embryo or fetus from the top of its head to the bottom of the torso (**Figure 2a**). Popularly called the Robinson's CRL curve, it is the most accurate estimation of gestational age in early pregnancy, owing to the little biological variability at that time. Thus, CRL measurement has become the universal pregnancy dating tool to avoid the last menstrual date recall error [11, 12]. If the GA is >14 weeks then head circumference (HC) is used for dating the pregnancy (**Figure 2b**).

3.1.1.1.2.2 Diagnose multiple pregnancies and determination of chorionicity

Overall, twin pregnancies are at higher risk than singleton pregnancies for aneuploidy. This is mostly due to advanced maternal age in twin pregnancies. Determination of chorionicity of a twin pregnancy is of paramount importance, and the first trimester assessment has a better accuracy rate of 96–100% versus approximately 80% in the second trimester [16–19]. Chorionicity, rather than zygosity, has a major impact on the outcome of twin pregnancies mainly because of specific complications secondary to placental anastomoses, such as twin-to-twin transfusion syndrome (TTTS), selective fetal growth restriction (sFGR), twin anemia polycythemia sequence (TAPS), twin reversed arterial perfusion (TRAP) [20, 21]. The presence of the lambda sign (due to the interposed chorionic tissue) (**Figure 3a**) is suggestive of DCDA twins and the presence of the T sign is suggestive of MCDA twins (**Figure 3b**).

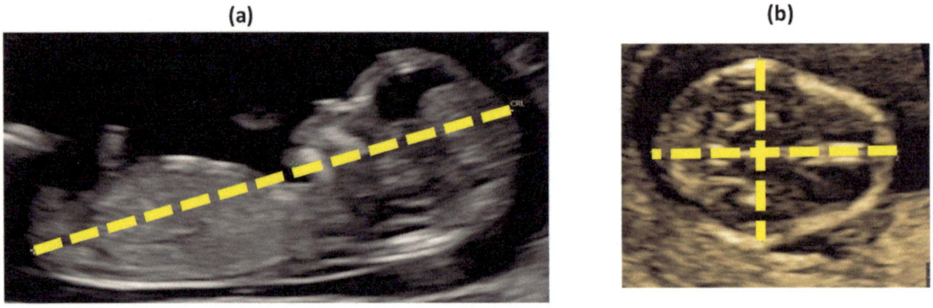

Figure 2.
Dating parameters. (a) Midsagittal plane of a fetus showing measurement of -rump length (CRL)-dating parameter <14 weeks GA, (b) measurement of head circumference (HC)-dating parameter >14 weeks GA.

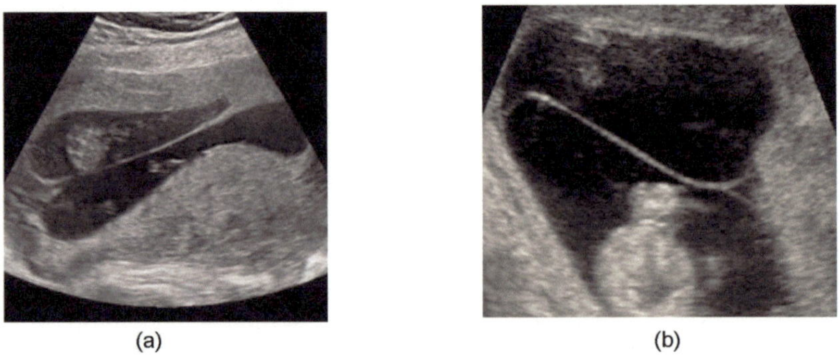

Figure 3.
Assessment of chorionicity. (a) Lambda sign-DCDA twins, (b) T sign-MCDA twins.

3.1.1.1.2.3 Identification of aneuploidy markers

Nuchal translucency (NT) is a subcutaneous collection of fluid between the skin and soft tissue overlying the fetal spine at the back of the neck in the sagittal plane. It is the most important marker used in the first trimester for aneuploidy risk calculation. This was demonstrated by Nicolaides in the early 1990s and was found to be strongly associated with fetal aneuploidy [22, 23]. Increased NT is associated with trisomy 21/13/18, Turner syndrome and other chromosomal defects, fetal structural malformations, and genetic syndromes. Though NT tends to resolve, it can evolve into increased nuchal fold thickness or cystic hygromas with or without hydrops. **Figure 4a** and **b** is representative of normal and increased nuchal translucency, respectively.

NT must be accurately imaged and measured in a reproducible way following the standards put forth by the Fetal Medicine Foundation and Perinatal Quality Foundation for aneuploidy detection to be accurate. The optimal gestational age for measurement of fetal NT is 11–13 + 6 weeks when the fetal CRL is between 45 and 84 mm. Measurement is done in the sagittal plane with the neck in a neutral position, and the image is magnified so that the screen is filled with the fetal head, neck, and upper thorax. The calipers are placed on the inner borders of the widest aspect of the nuchal space, perpendicular to the long axis of the fetus, with the horizontal crossbar within the space [24]. Though there is no clarity in the definition of increased NT beyond the cutoff of 3.5 mm, NT is said to be increased when it is >99th centile for the CRL or > 1.9 MOM for the measured CRL [25]. The causes of increased NT [23, 26] are cardiac defects and dysfunction, venous congestion in the head and neck, the altered composition of the extracellular matrix, failure of lymphatic drainage, fetal anemia, fetal hypoproteinemia, and fetal infection [26].

3.1.1.1.2.4 Other aneuploidy markers

3.1.1.1.2.4.1 Heart rate

In normal pregnancy, the fetal heart rate (FHR) increases from about 100 bpm at 5 weeks of gestation to 170 bpm at 10 weeks and then decreases to 155 bpm by 14 weeks. Between 11 and 14 weeks, trisomy 13 and Turner syndrome are associated with tachycardia, whereas bradycardia is noted in trisomy 18 and triploidy. Inclusion

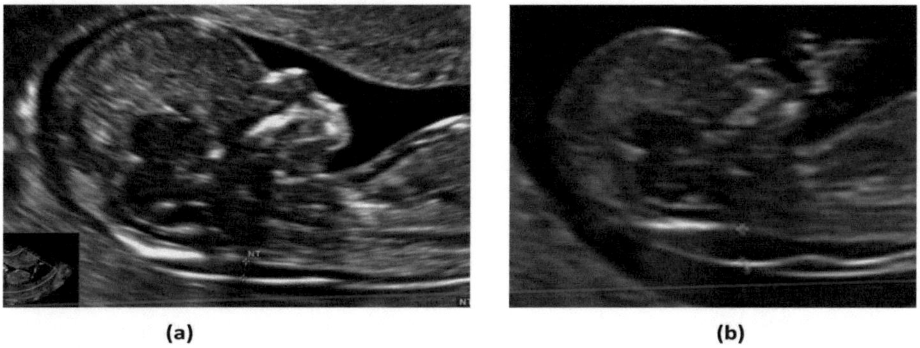

Figure 4.
Measurement of nuchal translucency (NT). (a) Sagittal section of fetus showing normal nuchal translucency—1.8 mm, (b) sagittal section of fetus showing increased nuchal translucency—4.1 mm.

of FHR is important in differentiating trisomy 18 and 13, which in other respects show common features like increased fetal NT and decreased maternal serum free B hCG and PAPP-A [26].

3.1.1.1.2.4.2 Nasal bone

Nasal bone (NB) assessment is done between 11 and 13 + 6 weeks when the CRL is between 45 and 84 mm. In the midsagittal view of the fetal profile, NB is imaged as three distinct lines. The top line represents the skin and the bottom one, which is thicker and more echogenic than the overlying skin, represents the NB. A third line, almost in continuity with the skin, but at a higher level, represents the tip of the nose. At 11–13 + 6 weeks the NB is absent in 1–3% of euploid fetuses, 60% of fetuses with trisomy 21, 50% of fetuses with trisomy18, and 40% of fetuses with trisomy 13. Assessment of the NB improves the performance of combined screening, increasing the detection rate from 90% to 93% and decreasing the false positive rate from 5% to 3% [26]. **Figure 5a** and **b** shows the ossified and unossified nasal bone, respectively.

3.1.1.1.2.4.3 Tricuspid regurgitation (TR)

TR assessment is done between 11 and 13 + 6 weeks when the CRL measures 45–84 mm. No regurgitation should be noted across the fetal tricuspid valve during

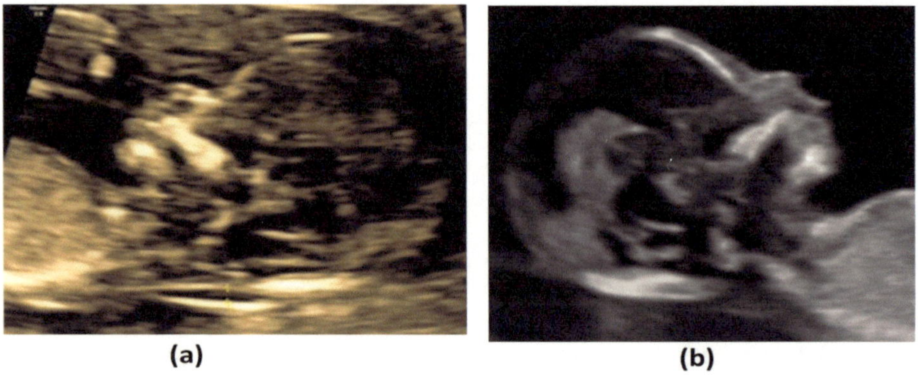

Figure 5.
Assessment of NB. (a) NB—seen as the bottom line, (b) unossified nasal bone—absence of bottom line.

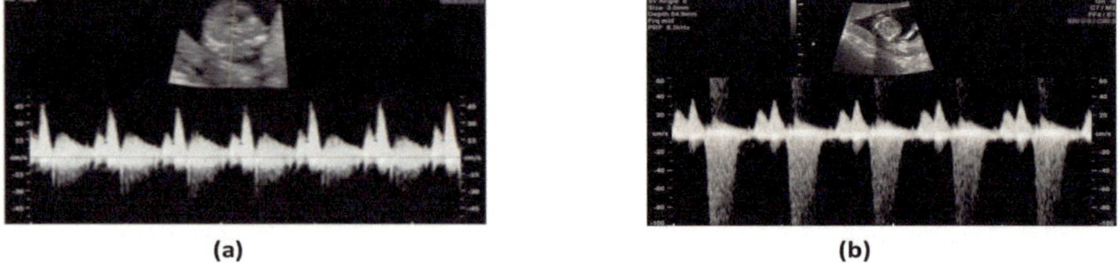

Figure 6.
Assessment of tricuspid flow. (a) Axial section of the fetal thorax with spectral wave Doppler imaging showing normal flow pattern across the tricuspid valve, (b) axial section of the fetal thorax with spectral wave Doppler flow showing tricuspid regurgitation.

systole. Regurgitation is significant if it occurs in more than half of systole with a velocity of more than 60 cm/s and is noted in about 1% of euploid fetuses, 55% of fetuses with trisomy 21, and 30% in fetuses with trisomy 18 and trisomy 13. **Figure 6a** and **b** shows normal tricuspid flow pattern and tricuspid regurgitation, respectively. Assessment of the tricuspid flow improves the detection rate from 90% to 95% and decreases the false positive rate from 3% to 2.5%. If there is tricuspid regurgitation, it is pertinent that a detailed cardiac evaluation is done to diagnose or exclude major cardiac defects [26].

3.1.1.1.2.4.4 Ductus venosus flow

The ductus venosus is a short trumpet-shaped vessel that shunts oxygenated blood preferentially to the fetal heart. It has a triphasic pattern and the forward 'a wave corresponds to the atrial systole. Reversed a wave in ductus venosus is associated with an increased risk for chromosomal abnormalities, cardiac defects, and fetal death. At 11–13 + 6 weeks, abnormal ductal flow is observed in 5% of chromosomally normal fetuses and about 80% of fetuses with trisomy 21. Assessment of ductus venosus improves the performance of combined screening, increasing the detection rate from 90% to 95% and decreasing the false positive rate from 3% to 2.5%. Though in 80% of cases with isolated reversed a wave the pregnancy outcome is normal, a detailed cardiac evaluation should be done to rule out cardiac defects in fetuses with an a-wave reversal in ductus venosus (**Figure 7a** and **b**) [26]'.

3.1.1.1.2.5 Identification of structural anomalies

There has been a paradigm shift from the identification of fetal aneuploidies in the 1980s to the early identification of structural/genetic abnormalities due to innovation in USG imaging technology. The commonly identified anomalies are given below: Acrania, alobar holoprosencephaly, body stalk anomaly, omphalocele, megacystis, and early hydrops. **Figure 8a–f** depicts these commonly diagnosed first trimester anomalies.

3.1.1.1.3 Biochemical screening/risk assessment.

Every pregnant woman has a background or apriori risk to bear a fetus with aneuploidy. This is based on her age and history of aneuploidy. The risk for trisomies increases with maternal age, but Turner syndrome and triploidy do not change with maternal age. The patient-specific risk is calculated by multiplying the apriori risk

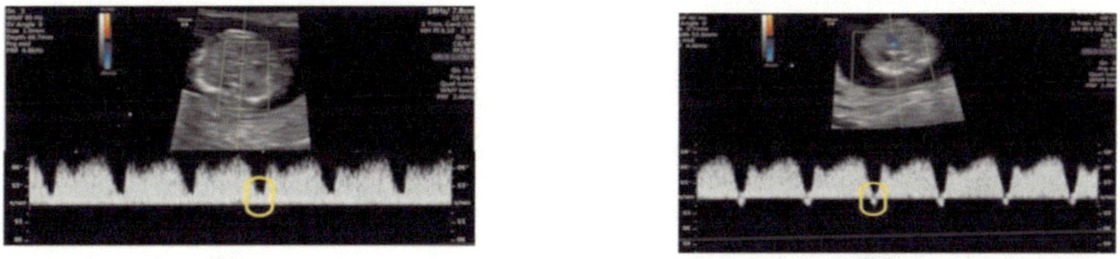

(a) (b)

Figure 7.
Assessment of ductus venosus (DV) flow. (a) Axial section of the fetal abdomen with spectral wave Doppler flow showing normal ductus venosus flow with normal 'a' wave, (b) axial section of the fetal abdomen with spectral wave Doppler flow showing abnormal ductus venosus flow with reversed 'a' wave.

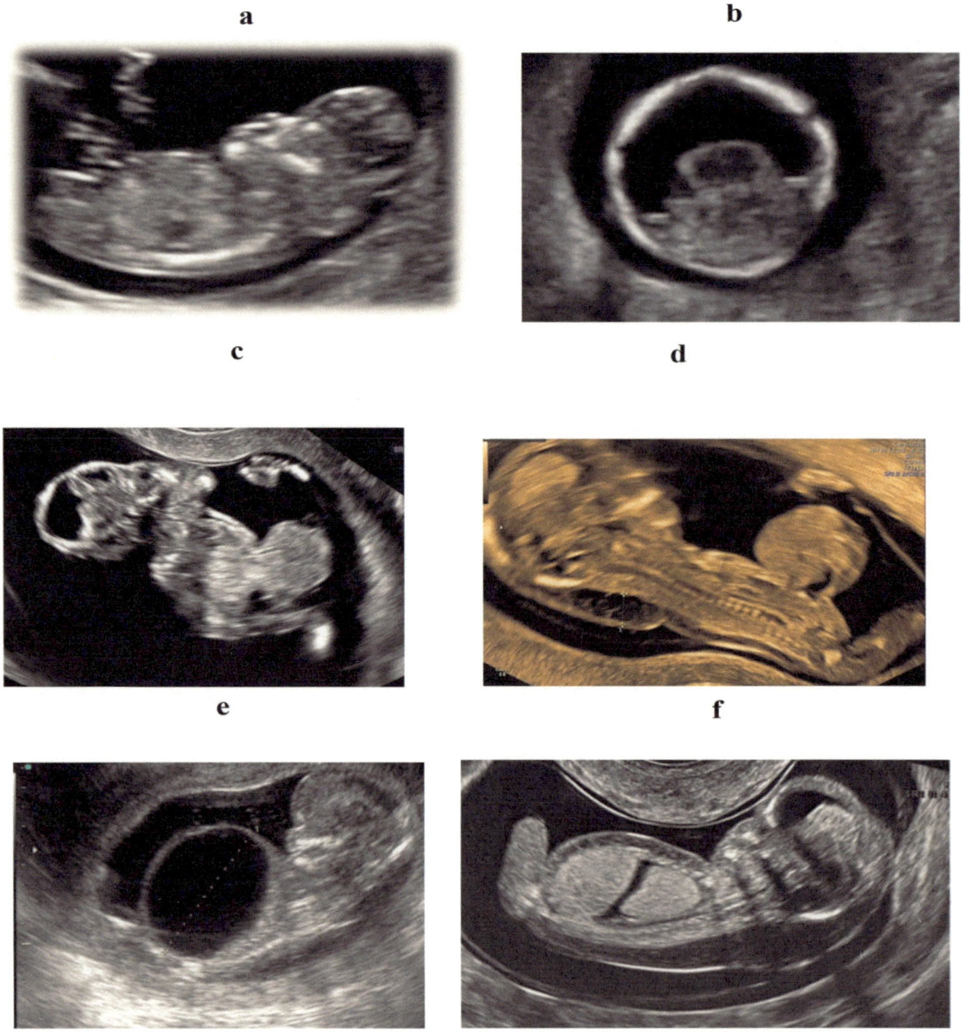

Figure 8.
Commonly identified anomalies in the first trimester. (a) Acrania, (b) alobar holoprosencephaly, (c) body stalk anomaly, (d) omphalocele, (e) megacystis, (f) early hydrops.

with a composite likelihood ratio, which is obtained from the screening tests performed during the pregnancy in the first and second trimesters. Each time a test is carried out the apriori risk is multiplied by the likelihood ratio of the test to calculate a new risk, which subsequently becomes the apriori risk for the next test.

Aneuploid pregnancies are associated with altered maternal serum concentrations of various fetoplacental products, namely HCG and PAPPA. First trimester combined screening integrates nuchal translucency with maternal serum HCG and PAPPA. HCG assay can be either intact HCG or free beta unit of HCG depending on the local laboratory guidelines and clinical practice, albeit the two are considered comparable [23]. Individual analytes are converted to multiples of the median (MOM) adjusting for maternal age, maternal weight, smoking status, ethnicity, and gestational age. The pattern of increase or decrease in analyte levels affects the risk for trisomies 21, 18, and 13 and at a predetermined value the test is deemed positive or abnormal. For

Maternal	Fetal
Risk stratification into high/low risk if not done already	Determine the age of the fetus
Identify women who need additional care	Assess chorionicity in twins and higher-order multiples
Screening for preeclampsia	Screening for aneuploidies/anomalies
Screening for preterm labor	Screening for small for gestational age (SGA)

Table 1.
Indications of 11–14 weeks assessment.

trisomy 21, this is often presented as a first trimester risk of 1:250 and for trisomy 18 and trisomy 13, a cut-off of 1:150 is used (**Table 1**).

In euploid pregnancies, the average maternal serum HCG is 1.0 MOM and PAPP-A is 1.0 MOM. In trisomy 21 pregnancies, maternal serum HCG is increased by twofold and PAPP-A is reduced to half compared to normal pregnancies. In trisomies 18 and 13, maternal serum HCG and PAPP-A are decreased. In cases of sex chromosomal anomalies, maternal serum HCG is normal and PAPP-A is low. In paternally derived triploidy, maternal serum free HCG is greatly increased, whereas PAPP-A is mildly decreased. Maternally derived triploidy is associated with markedly decreased maternal serum HCG and PAPP-A [26, 27]. **Table 2** depicts the analyte levels in various fetal trisomies in the first trimester and screening by a combination of fetal NT and maternal serum PAPP-A and HCG can identify about 90% of all these chromosomal abnormalities for a false positive rate of 5% [26, 27]. **Table 3** depicts the detection rates and false positive rates of various combinations of screening tools and markers used in the first trimester [26].

Analytes	Trisomy 21	Trisomy 18/ T13	Paternally derived triploidy (Type I)	Maternally derived triploidy (Type 2)
NT	Increased	Increased	Increased	Normal
HCG	Increased	Decreased	Marked increase	Marked decrease
PAPPA	Decreased	Decreased	Mild decrease	Marked decrease

Table 2.
Multiple marker levels associated with trisomies in the first trimester.

Screening tool	Detection rate (%)	False positive rate (%)
Age	30	5
NT alone	60	5
Combined (NT + biochemistry)	85–90	5
NT + NB	90	5
NT + NB + biochemistry	95	3
NT + NB + DVflow + TR + biochemistry	95–96	2–3

Table 3.
Detection and false positive rates of different combinations of screening tools and markers used in the first trimester. Modified from [26].

As the biochemical analytes (HCG and PAPPA) are increased twofold in twin pregnancies, the performance of combined screening is 15% lower when compared to singleton pregnancies [28].

3.1.1.1.4 Posttest counseling

Posttest counseling is mandatory for any screening program. When a positive or negative screening test result is obtained, the patient should be counseled regarding the adjusted likelihood of carrying a fetus with the aneuploidies evaluated and a diagnostic test is offered. The possibility for the fetus to be affected by genetic disorders which are not evaluated by the screening or diagnostic test should also be reviewed. In the event of a prenatal diagnosis of fetal aneuploidy, the patient and family should be counseled appropriately so that she can make informed decisions regarding further pregnancy management.

3.1.1.2 Second trimester screening

The triple screen which includes the analytes alpha feto protein (AFP), HCG, and serum estriol has a poor detection rate of 60% and was used in the 1980s. The quadruple test which was formulated by the addition of dimeric inhibin A to the triple screen in the 1990s replaced it and is the only current second trimester multiple marker screening tests widely used. A quadruple screen is performed between 15 and 21 weeks when the Biparietal diameter (BPD) is between 34 and 52 mm, the measurement varying between labs. The pattern of change in analytes is depicted in **Table 4** [29].

Since the early 2000s, the quadruple test detection rate is 81–83% at a 5% false positive rate in two large prospective trials- the Serum, Urine, and Ultrasound Screening Study (SURUSS) [24] and the First and Second Trimester Evaluation of Risk (FASTER) [10] trials.

As the second trimester quadruple marker screening offers no advantage over first trimester screening, it is used only if first trimester screening is unavailable in certain settings or if the antenatal woman books too late to receive first trimester screening.

3.1.1.3 Combination of first and second trimester screening

This is based on the concept that aneuploidy detection will be significantly increased if first trimester biochemistry and nuchal translucency screening is combined with a second trimester quadruple marker test. However, these two tests should not be done as independent tests as it increases the false positive rate thus making counseling difficult. There are two different methods of screening—integrated test

Analytes	Trisomy 21	Trisomy 18
AFP	Decreased	Decreased
Estriol	Decreased	Decreased
HCG	Increased	Decreased
Inhibin	Increased	Not applicable

Table 4.
Multiple marker levels associated with trisomies in the second trimester.

and sequential screening, which are further subdivided into stepwise and contingent sequential screening.

Integrated screening involves testing the first trimester serum analytes (HCG and PAPPA) and NT at 11–14 weeks followed by quadruple screening between 15 and 21 weeks of GA and a single risk is calculated. This integrated approach has a 94% sensitivity in detecting T21 and 93% detection of T18 [30] and the result was abnormal in 93% of cases with trisomy 13, in 91% with triploidy, and 80% with monosomy. Serum integrated screening is done when NT is unavailable and only the biochemistry is taken into consideration. This has a detection rate of 85–88% for T21 at a 5% false positive rate [24].

In sequential screening, first trimester screening with nuchal translucency and serum analytes is performed and the patient is informed about the results based on the understanding that, if the risk exceeds a predetermined cut-off (≥1 in 30), she will be offered diagnostic testing. There are two types of sequential screening. With stepwise sequential screening, women at high risk in the first trimester are offered diagnostic testing and the rest go on to complete the quadruple marker screening in the second trimester, after which the women who are screen positive are offered diagnostic testing and the rest are reassured and no further testing is indicated. Based on data from the FASTER trial, stepwise sequential screening using a first trimester risk cut-off of 1:30 and an overall cut-off of 1:270 yielded a 92% trisomy 21 detection rate at a 5% false positive rate [24]. In contingent sequential screening, after women at high risk are offered a diagnostic test, the remaining women are divided into two groups. The lowest risk women (<1:1500) are reassured and receive no further screening, whereas those at intermediate risk (1 in 270 to 1 in 1500) are followed up with quadruple marker screening. Based on data from the FASTER trial, the trisomy 21 detection rate was 91% with the contingent screening at a 5% false positive rate [24].

3.1.2 Cell-free–based DNA screening

Noninvasive prenatal screening (NIPS) or cell-free–based DNA screening was introduced into the armamentarium of aneuploidy screening in 2011. This test identifies circulating DNA fragments that are primarily placental in origin, from apoptotic trophoblasts. Assaying of cell-free DNA is done in three ways for aneuploidy screening: whole-genome sequencing (massive parallel shotgun sequencing-MPSS); chromosome selective sequencing (targeted); and single nucleotide polymorphism analysis (SNP). It can be performed after 9–10 weeks of gestation, and the turnaround time of the results is within 7–10 days. The detection rate is 99% for trisomy 21, 96% for trisomy 18, and approximately 90% for trisomy 13 and monosomy X [8, 9]. According to a meta-analysis of 37 studies of cell-free DNA screening in high-risk pregnancies, the pooled sensitivity to detect trisomy 21 was 99.2% (95% confidence interval 98.5–99.6%), and the specificity was 99.9%, and the false positive rate was only 0.1% [29, 31]. Detection rates of trisomies 18 and 13 are 96% and 91%, respectively, each with a specificity of 99.9%. For detection of monosomy X (Turner syndrome), the sensitivity of cell-free DNA was approximately 90% with a specificity of 99.8% [29, 31–35]. **Table 5** depicts the different characteristics, the detection rates, the false positive rates, and the positive predictive values of the different screening tests to detect T21 [29].

The high PPV of cell-free DNA screening is dependent on maternal age at delivery which means in younger women, a positive screening test result is more likely to be falsely positive regardless of the aneuploidy. For a woman in her early 20s, the PPV

Screening test for T21	Sensitivity %	False positive rate %	Positive predictive value %
First trimester screening (NT + biochemistry)	80–84	5	3–4
Triple screen	69	5	2
Quadruple screening	80–82	5	3
Serum integrated test	85–88	4.9	5
Fully integrated test	94–96	5	5
Stepwise sequential	92	5.1	5
Contingent sequential	91	4.5	5
Cell-free DNA	99	0.1	48–98 (for ages 20–45 respectively)

Table 5.
Characteristics and performance of different screening tests [29].

may be close to 50% for fetal trisomy 21, but this percentage is considerably higher in older women, which is clinically relevant while counseling before cell-free DNA screening considering the expensive nature of the test [29].

As the placenta and the fetus do not share the same chromosomal content, false positives can occur especially when there is confined placental mosaicism (CPM) and a vanishing co-twin with an identifiable fetal pole. Hence cell-free DNA screening is not recommended in such conditions [36, 37]. Moreover, as this screening examines the maternal DNA, rare cases of maternal mosaicism and malignancy have also been identified [38, 39] by the presence of more than one aneuploidies in the test. Another disadvantage of this screening method is the 'No Call' result which is seen in 4–5% of screened pregnancies. This is due to a reduced fetal fraction of less than 4% which is seen in lower gestational age, obese women, small placentation, and aneuploidies [40–42]. If a no-call result is reported the patient should be counseled by a geneticist in detail regarding the possible cause and is offered a repeat test or invasive amniocentesis keeping in mind the high chance of no-call in the repeat test which is as high as 40%.

Traditional screening	Cell-free DNA screening
First-line screening in low-risk pregnancies	Can be considered as first-line in high-risk pregnancies A secondary screening if the traditional screen is positive
Accurate GA is essential	Done any time after 10 weeks GA
85–94% sensitivity	99% sensitivity
5% FPR	0.1% FPR
Soft markers are used to modify the risk	Soft markers are not used to modify the risk
Screen positive results may include other chromosomal abnormalities not detected with cell-free DNA	When used as a secondary screening test, does not diagnose other aneuploidies other than T21, 18, 13, 45X, 47 XXX, XXY, and XYY

Table 6.
Comparison of traditional and cell-free DNA screening [29].

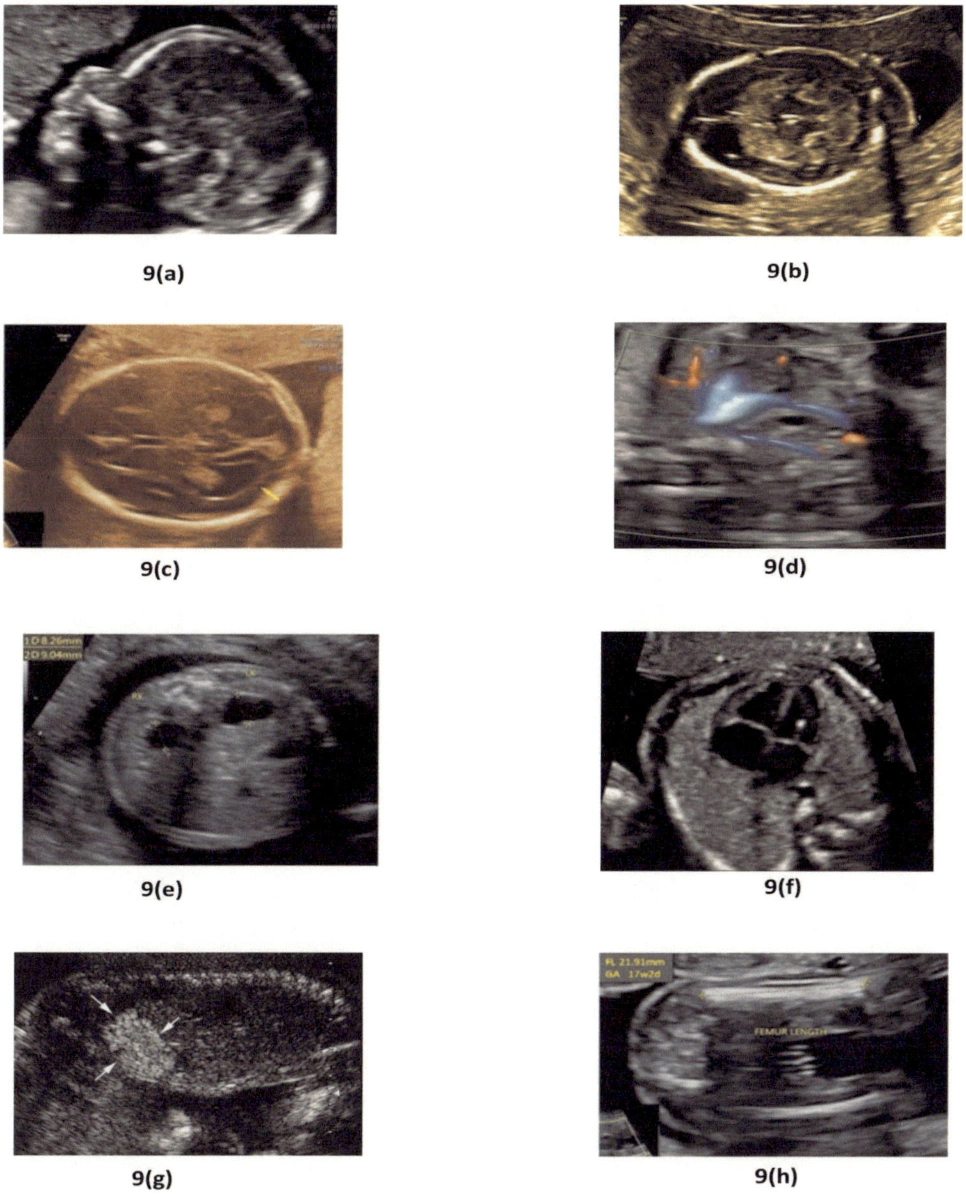

Figure 9.
Commonly noted second trimester USG soft markers. (a) Profile view of the fetal face showing unossified nasal bone (UNB), (b) transcerebellar plane showing increased nuchal fold thickness (NFT), (c) fetal transventricular plane showing ventriculomegaly, (d) axial section of fetal thorax showing aberrant right subclavian artery (ARSA), (e) axial section of the fetal abdomen showing bilateral renal pelviectasis, (f) axial section of fetal thorax showing echogenic cardiac focus in the left ventricle, (g) sagittal view of abdomen showing fetal bowel as echogenic as surrounding bone, (h) short femur length corresponding to 17 weeks in a fetus at 19 weeks of gestation.

Because of its high detection and low false positive rate, cell-free DNA screening may be offered as either a primary screen or secondary screening test to women who test positive on a traditional screening test before proceeding with a diagnostic test. If an abnormal traditional screening result is followed by a normal cell-free DNA screen, the risk for a chromosomal abnormality is approximately 2% [43]. However, the time required for cell-free DNA screening (7–10 days) may delay aneuploidy diagnosis to the point that pregnancy termination may no longer be an option for those who choose it. Because of the above-mentioned limitations and the reduced cost-effectiveness in low-risk pregnancies, traditional screening tests are still considered the choice of first-line screening for low-risk pregnancies [8]. However, cell-free DNA screening is recommended as a screening option in advanced maternal age (maternal age > 35 years at delivery), high/intermediate-risk in traditional screening, presence of an ultrasonographic soft marker, prior pregnancy with h/o trisomy, or known carrier of a balanced Robertsonian translocation involving chromosomes 21, 13, and 14 [9]. Currently, cell-free DNA screening detects specific chromosomal abnormalities, namely trisomy 21, 18, and 13; 45, X; and 47 XXX, XXY, and XYY [44]. It should be noted that prenatal diagnosis is recommended whenever an aneuploidy screening test is abnormal and pregnancy termination should not be based on the results of any screening test. A comparison of traditional and cell-free DNA screening is given in **Table 6**. Cell-free DNA is not offered if the first trimester scan reveals any structural abnormalities.

3.1.2.1 Role of USG in the second trimester (to rule out anomalies and evaluate for soft markers)

We have already elaborately learned about the role of USG in the first trimester. Targeted imaging of fetus for anomalies (TIFFA) is a level 2 USG done at 18–24 weeks depending on the local protocols. There is a role for targeted scan after a positive aneuploidy testing as the presence of an abnormality or multiple soft markers increases the risk of aneuploidy by 50–60% [45]. It is also noted that 25–30% of fetuses with Down syndrome and almost all fetuses with T18/13 will have major abnormalities [46, 47]. Soft markers are normal USG variants with no/trivial clinical sequelae, are transient and resolve with advancing gestation or after birth, and are noted in 10% of euploid pregnancies. The most commonly noted second trimester soft

Soft marker	Description	Likelihood ratio
Ventriculomegaly	Lateral ventricular atrial measurement >10 mm	3.81
Thickened nuchal fold	Distance between the outer edge of the occipital bone to outer skin in transcerebellar diameter if >6 mm	3.79
Unossified nasal bone	Unossified nasal bone in the profile view of the fetal face	6.58
ARSA	The right subclavian artery arises directly from the aortic arch instead of originating from the brachiocephalic artery	3.94
Echogenic bowel	Fetal small bowel as echogenic as bone	1.65
ECF LV	Echogenic tissue in one or both ventricles of the heart seen on a standard 4 chamber view	0.95
Pelviectasis	Renal pelvis measuring >4 mm	1.08
Short femur	Measurement <5th percentile for gestational age	0.61
Short humerus	Measurement <5th percentile for gestational age	0.78

Table 7.
Various second trimester soft markers and their likelihood ratios.

markers are unossified/hypoplastic NB, ventriculomegaly, increased nuchal skinfold thickness, aberrant right subclavian artery, echogenic intracardiac focus, echogenic bowel, pelviectasis, and short femur or humerus length. When a marker has been identified, the posttest odds for trisomy 21 are derived by multiplying the pretest odds (obtained by first/second trimester screening) by the positive LR for each detected marker. The images of various second trimester soft markers are depicted in **Figure 9a–h**. Metaanalysis by Agathakleous et al. in 2013 suggested that when the targeted anomaly scan reveals no abnormalities and soft markers then the aneuploidy risk is reduced by 7.7-fold. **Table 7** shows the various markers and their likelihood ratios [48].

3.1.2.2 Diagnostic tests of aneuploidy

Diagnostic testing allows patients to know with certainty whether the pregnancy is affected by a particular genetic condition. Abnormal screening tests in the first or second trimester must be followed up by diagnostic tests before any final decisions are made. Commonly performed diagnostic tests include chorionic villus sampling (**Figure 10**), and amniocentesis (**Figure 11**). Preimplantation genetic diagnosis is considered in known cases of familial syndromes or previously affected children with

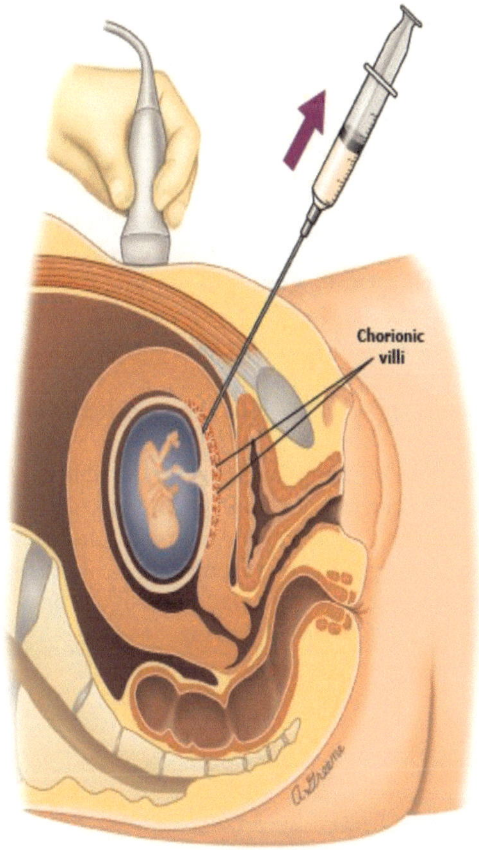

Figure 10.
Transabdominal chorionic villus sampling.

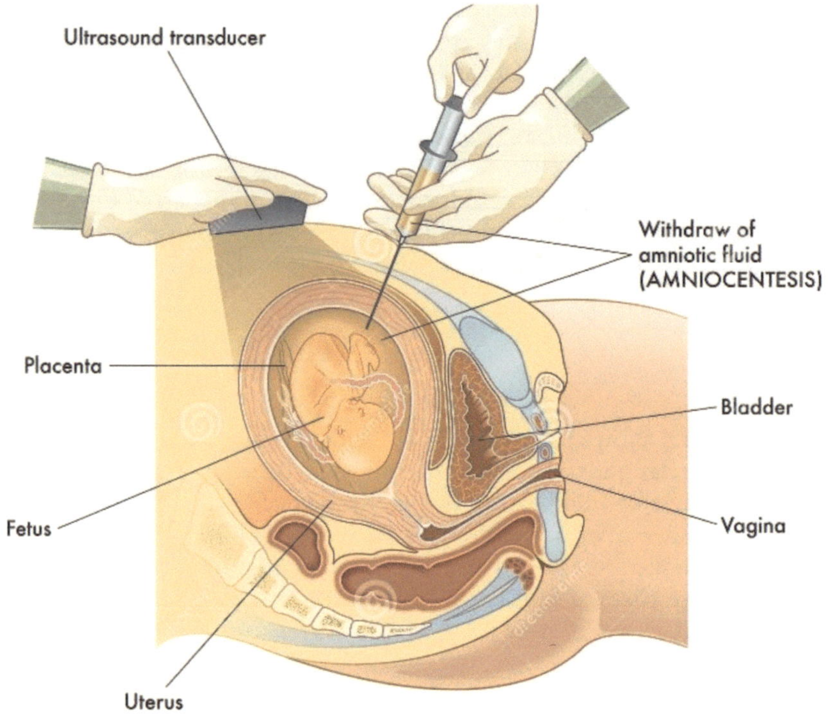

Figure 11.
Amniocentesis.

parents being carriers. Rapid aneuploidy testing using either quantitative fluorescent polymerase chain reaction (qfPCR) or fluorescent in-situ hybridization (FISH), will detect the major trisomies (13, 18, and 21) and Turners syndrome (45XO) and the results are issued in 1–3 working days. Full karyotyping is then performed following culturing of the cells. This takes 10–14 days and involves microscopic examination of cells and can detect other chromosomal rearrangements. However, as this approach will not detect very small submicroscopic changes, known as copy number variations (CNVs), chromosomal microarray (CMA) has replaced conventional karyotyping in identifying the CNVs.

The advantage of prenatal diagnosis is that when an anomaly or a genetic disease is diagnosed prenatally, it helps the obstetrician and neonatologist to counsel the family, discuss the available options, and to initiate a neonatal management plan even before delivery of the fetus. In certain cases, treatment may be instituted in utero. Although diagnostic testing is recommended to be available to all women, regardless of maternal age, patients should be counseled regarding types of invasive procedures, including the expected benefits, risks, and technical aspects of the test.

The indications of diagnostic testing are as follows:

1. Positive screening test for common trisomies.

2. Previous pregnancy complicated by fetal trisomy.

3. At least one major or two minor fetal structural anomalies in the current pregnancy abnormalities.

4. A desire to have the most reliable information about the fetal karyotype.

5. A desire to have a comprehensive genetic analysis that will detect both autosomal and sex chromosome aneuploidy and pathological copy number variants.

3.1.2.3 Chorionic villus sampling (CVS)

CVS is the only diagnostic test available in the first trimester and allows for diagnostic analyses, including quantitative Fluorescent Polymerase Chain Reaction (qFPCR), karyotype, microarray, molecular testing, and gene sequencing. CVS is performed between 10 and 14 weeks of gestation. Early CVS which was performed before 9 weeks in the past is no longer recommended as it is shown to increase the risk of limb deformities and oromandibular malformations.

Under ultrasonographic guidance, a sample of placental tissue is collected for genetic evaluation through a catheter placed through either the transcervical or transabdominal route without entering the sac (**Figure 10**). CVS allows for earlier prenatal diagnosis and earlier pregnancy termination if desired. A disadvantage of CVS is confined placental mosaicism (CPM) which is noted in 1–2% of CVS results. Pregnancy loss attributed to CVS is approximately 1 in 450 according to recent data [49–51].

3.1.2.4 Amniocentesis

Amniocentesis is a technique by which amniotic fluid is withdrawn from the amniotic sac using a needle under continuous ultrasound guidance via a transabdominal approach to obtain a sample of fetal exfoliated cells, transudates, urine, or secretions. It can be performed from 16 weeks of pregnancy onwards (**Figure 11**). The various tests which can be performed in the amniotic sample are chromosomal, biochemical, molecular, and microbial studies, the most common being prenatal diagnosis of chromosomal abnormalities, single-gene disorders, and fetal infection The procedure has a risk of fetal loss of approximately 0.5% (range, 0.06–1%) [50, 51].

3.1.2.5 Preimplantation genetic diagnosis

Preimplantation genetic diagnosis (PGD) is a test to detect the abnormality before embryo transfer so that only unaffected embryos are transferred to the patient. This helps in the earlier detection of chromosomal and genetic abnormalities. After in vitro fertilization (IVF) a polar body or a single cell from the blastocyst is removed and examined for aneuploidies/genetic disorders (**Figure 12**). However, it is recommended that all pregnancies conceived with IVF/PGD should be offered confirmatory testing with CVS or amniocentesis as false negative reports are possible [52, 53].

3.2 Preeclampsia/SGA screening

Prediction of PE and SGA can be done in the first trimester by a combination of maternal demographic characteristics, uterine artery pulsatility index (Ut art PI), mean arterial pressure (MAP), and maternal serum biochemical markers serum PAPP-A and PlGF [54].

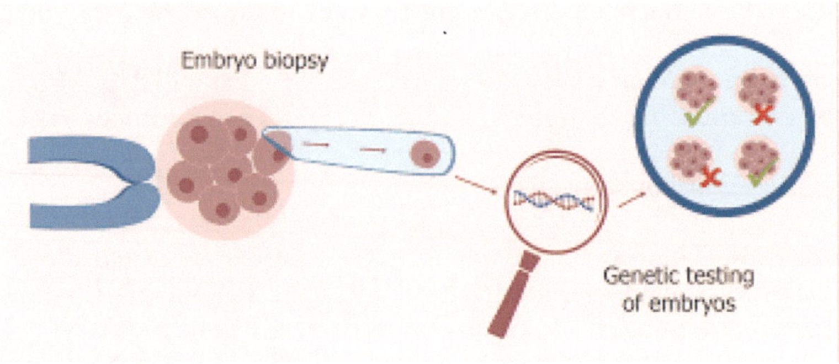

Figure 12.
Preimplantation genetic diagnosis.

SGA is defined as birth weight below the 10th centile for the gestational age though there are cutoffs varying between the 3rd and 10th centile. The prevalence of SGA is estimated to be 8–11%. The SGA babies are prone to develop complications like prematurity, neonatal asphyxia, hypothermia, hypoglycemia, hyperbilirubinemia, hypocalcemia, polycythemia, sepsis, and death [54]; and long-term morbidities like learning difficulties, cognitive, and behavioral defects.

Preeclampsia (PE) is a multisystem disorder of pregnancy [55, 56] and develops in 2–5% of pregnant women and is one of the leading causes of maternal and perinatal morbidity and mortality [57, 58]. The International Society for the Study of Hypertension in Pregnancy (ISSHP) definition is the accepted one by international bodies, [59] which defines gestational hypertension as systolic blood pressure (SBP) at ≥140 mm Hg and/or diastolic blood pressure (DBP) at ≥90 mm Hg on at least two occasions measured 4 h apart developing after 20 weeks of gestation in previously normotensive women. PE is defined as gestational hypertension accompanied by ≥1 of the following conditions at or after 20 weeks of gestation: (a) Proteinuria (≥30 mg/mol protein: creatinine ratio; ≥300 mg/24 h; or ≥ 2 + dipstick) (b) Maternal organ dysfunction, including acute kidney injury (creatinine ≥90 μmol/L; 1 mg/dL) liver involvement (elevated transaminases, e.g. alanine aminotransferase or aspartate aminotransferase >40 IU/L) with or without right upper quadrant or epigastric abdominal pain, neurological complications (e.g. eclampsia, altered mental status, blindness, stroke, clonus, severe headaches, and persistent visual scotomata) or hematological complications (thrombocytopenia—platelet count <150,000/μL) or c) uteroplacental dysfunction (fetal growth restriction, abnormal umbilical artery Doppler waveform analysis, or stillbirth).

PE can be further subclassified into [59]:

1. Early-onset PE (with delivery <34 weeks GA)

2. Preterm PE (with delivery <37 weeks GA)

3. Late-onset PE (with delivery ≥34 weeks GA)

4. Term PE (with delivery ≥37 weeks GA)

Most common maternal complications include placental abruption, HELLP syndrome, acute pulmonary edema, respiratory distress syndrome, acute renal failure, intracranial hemorrhage, and death [60, 61]. The early perinatal complications are fetal growth restriction, nonreassuring FHR during labor, oligohydramnios, intrauterine fetal death (IUFD) preterm birth, low Apgar scores, need for NICU admission, and long-term complications are cerebral palsy, hearing loss, visual impairment, insulin resistance, diabetes mellitus, coronary artery disease, and hypertension.

Thus, the occurrence of PE and SGA contributes significantly to adverse pregnancy outcomes. Hence screening at 11–14 weeks GA, is of paramount importance as one can identify the patients prone to develop these disorders, prevent them to a considerable extent by starting on prophylactic Aspirin and be prepared to tackle the maternal and perinatal morbidity associated with it.

Maternal risk factors for PE and SGA prediction are nulliparity, age ≥ 40 years, BMI ≥35 kg/ m^2, family history of PE, interpregnancy interval > 10 years, hypertensive disease in a previous pregnancy, chronic hypertension, chronic renal disease, diabetes mellitus, or autoimmune disease [62]. Based on the history and presence of risk factors, the detection rate is only 39% for preterm PE and 34% for term PE at a 10.3% false positive rate. Thus, though history-based screening is useful in identifying at-risk women in clinical practice, it is not a sufficient tool for the effective prediction of PE.

Combined risk assessment for both early PE and preterm SGA is based on maternal characteristics, assessment of biophysical markers like MAP, uterine artery pulsatility index (UTPI), and biochemical markers, namely placental growth factor (PLGF) and PAPPA.

3.2.1 Measurement of mean arterial pressure (MAP)

MAP should be measured by validated automated and semiautomated devices. Women should be seated, with their arms well supported at the level of their heart and an appropriate-sized cuff should be used according to the mid-arm circumference (small, medium, or large). After resting for 5 min, blood pressure is recorded in both arms simultaneously and two sets of similar recordings are made at 1-minute intervals (**Figure 13**). The four sets of SBP and DBP measurements are included in the risk calculator and the final average MAP measurement is used for the calculation of patient-specific risk. The formula for the calculation of MAP is DBP + (SBP − DBP)/3 [63].

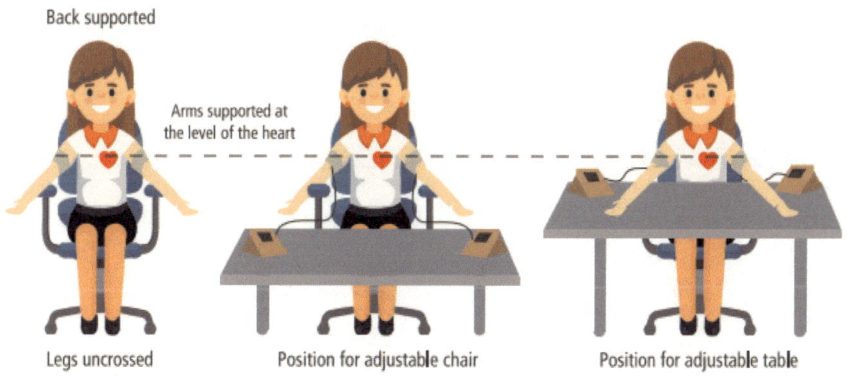

Figure 13.
Measurement of mean arterial pressure. Courtesy: Perkin Elmer life and analytical sciences (Wileyonline library.com).

3.2.2 Measurement of Uterine artery pulsatility Index (UTPI)

UTPI is measured along with an NT scan when the fetal CRL is between 45 and 84 mm and the GA between 11 and 13 + 6 weeks according to the criteria put forward by Fetal Medicine Foundation. For this measurement, a sagittal section of the uterus is obtained identifying the cervical canal and internal cervical os by transabdominal USG. Keeping the transducer in the midline and gentle tilting to both sides will identify each uterine artery in color flow mapping alongside the cervix at the level of the internal os. Pulsed-wave Doppler is then applied with the sampling gate at 2 mm to cover the whole vessel and the angle of insonation should be less than 30° (**Figure 14**). When three to five consecutive waveforms are obtained, the UTPI is measured and the mean UTPI of the left and right arteries is calculated [64, 65]. The first trimester abnormal UTPI is defined as greater than the 90th percentile, achieving a detection rate of 48%, at an 8% false positive rate, for the identification of early-onset PE. However, the detection rate for predicting late-onset PE reduces to 26% at a 7% false positive rate [64].

3.2.3 PLGF and PAPPA

PLGF and PAPPA are glycoproteins secreted by trophoblastic cells and changes in their levels have been implicated in the development of PE [66, 67]. Women who are prone to develop PE have significantly lower maternal PLGF and PAPPA concentrations in the first trimester than those with normal pregnancies. These biomarkers alone have a detection rate of 55% and 33%, respectively, at a 10% false positive rate, for the identification of both early and late-onset PE [68–71]. However, the detection rate with the combined approach is 90% for early PE, 75% for preterm PE, and 45% for term PE with a false positive rate of 10%. The detection rate of preterm SGA is 55% and term SGA is 44% with a false positive rate of 10%.

The ASPRE trial concluded that administration of low-dose aspirin, resulted in a 62% reduction in the incidence of preterm PE, when compared to placebo but did not have a significant reduction in the incidence of term PE [72]. However, it is pertinent to note that this combined first trimester screening of PE is less effective at predicting and preventing preeclampsia developing >37 weeks of gestation and hence the need for second trimester screening methods for PE.

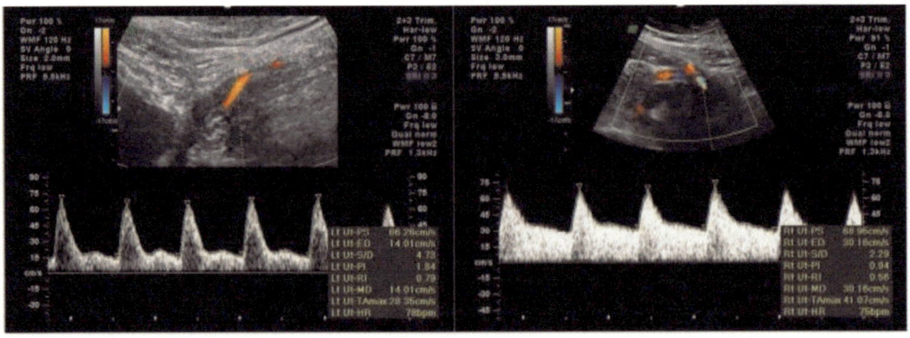

Figure 14.
Identification of the uterine artery at the level of the internal os and the demonstration of typical waveforms of the uterine artery Doppler in the first trimester of pregnancy.

3.2.4 Second trimester PE prediction

This is based on the concept that uteroplacental dysfunction occurs due to an imbalance in angiogenic and antiangiogenic factors. Circulating levels of the antiangiogenic protein, soluble fms-like tyrosine kinase-1 (sFlt-1) is increased, proangiogenic factor, PlGF is decreased and the sFlt-1/PlGF ratio is elevated before the onset of PE. Therefore, measurement of angiogenic markers, either alone or combined as part of the sFlt-1/PlGF ratio, has a significant value in preeclampsia prediction [73–75].

The prospective PROGNOSIS study [76], aimed to investigate the value of using the sFlt-1/PlGF ratio to predict the absence of PE within 1 week and to predict the presence of PE within 4 weeks in women with clinical suspicion of PE. sFlt-1/PlGF ratio cutoff of ≤38 was shown to have an NPV of 99.3% for ruling out development of PE within 1 week and a ratio > 38 demonstrated a PPV of 36.7% for ruling in preeclampsia within 4 weeks in a cohort of 700 women. The PPV for the occurrence of a combined endpoint of preeclampsia/eclampsia/HELLP syndrome, maternal and/or fetal adverse outcomes within 4 weeks was 65.5% [76]. Similar results were obtained in a separate study involving Asian women [77]. Thus, sFlt-1 and PlGF can be valuable biomarkers for the short-term prediction and detection of evolving preeclampsia in women with clinical signs and symptoms of the disorder, demonstrating a high NPV for ruling out preeclampsia, although the PPV remains relatively low. However, more research is needed to elucidate the benefits of the second trimester PE screening considering perinatal and maternal risk reduction and resource optimization.

Thus, the guideline to prevent PE is following the first trimester screening and assessment for preterm PE, women identified at high risk should receive aspirin prophylaxis commencing at 11–16 weeks of gestation at a dose of 150 mg to be taken every night until either 36 weeks of gestation, when delivery occurs, or when PE is diagnosed [78].

3.3 Screening for preterm labor

Approximately 11% of infants worldwide are born preterm, and the majority of cases occur in low-income countries [79]. Preterm birth (PTB) continues to be one of the leading causes of perinatal morbidity and mortality worldwide [80, 81]. Two-thirds of PTB cases are attributed to spontaneous PTB (SPTB) and the remaining one-third are medically indicated, due to maternal or fetal complications [82]. SPTB is defined as birth between 20 and 37 weeks of gestation following the spontaneous onset of labor, preterm prelabor rupture of membranes, or premature dilation of the cervix [83].

Preterm babies require prolonged hospitalization and are at high risk of adverse outcomes, including respiratory difficulty, necrotizing enterocolitis, feeding difficulties, blindness, deafness, intraventricular hemorrhage, higher risk of death at the age of 5 years, and neurodevelopmental sequelae when compared to their term counterparts [80, 84]. Thus, they need immense and prolonged health care, and hence for both the family and society PTB constitutes a major public health problem. Considering these issues, screening and early detection of pregnancies at the highest risk for SPTB will guide us in the implementation of management options and secondary prevention of morbidities associated with SPTB.

3.3.1 Identification of maternal risk factors

Demographic risk factors like African race, low socioeconomic status, and maternal characteristics like low BMI have been identified as poor risk factors with a relative risk (RR)—<2 in identifying women who are destined to develop SPTB. Other maternal risk factors are further subclassified into prior risk factors and pregnancy-specific risk factors. The prior risk factors are previous h/o preterm birth, a short interpregnancy interval of <6 months, family h/o preterm labor, congenital uterine malformations, infections of urinary and genital tracts, maternal smoking, and drug abuse. Pregnancy-specific risk factors are mid trimester short cervix <2.5 cm and bleeding per vaginum in the first or second trimester [82, 85]. Though the greatest risk factor for SPTB is a history of the previous SPTB, prediction of SPTB beyond that is very challenging considering the heterogeneous nature of risk factors and etiology.

3.3.2 USG screening

Universal cervical length screening is controversial due to its concern about cost-effectiveness and the possibility of unnecessary interventions. The most important risk factor for SPTB is a combination of short cervical length in a woman with previous h/o SPTB, which contributes to a relative risk of 3.3 [86, 87]. Cervical assessment is done by transvaginal ultrasound measurement of cervical length which is a safe, reliable, and highly reproducible tool when performed by trained providers [88]. In a mid trimester (16–24 weeks of gestation) scan, a cervical length of 2.5 cm corresponds to the 10th centile for the period of gestation, and hence if the transvaginal cervical length is <2.5 cm, it is considered to be short [89] (**Figure 15**). According to the guidelines put forth by the Society for Maternal-Fetal Medicine and the American College of Obstetricians and Gynecologists, serial cervical length surveillance is indicated for pregnant women with prior h/o SPTB from 16 to 24 weeks gestation though studies have shown that 82% of women who developed SPTB did not have a short cervical length during screening by transvaginal ultrasound [90].

3.3.3 Fetal fibronectin measurement

Fetal fibronectin (fFN) is an extracellular matrix glycoprotein that is present at the maternal-fetal interface of the amniotic membrane and is found in minimal quantity (<50 ng/ml) in the cervicovaginal secretions between 22 and 35 weeks of GA [91] and

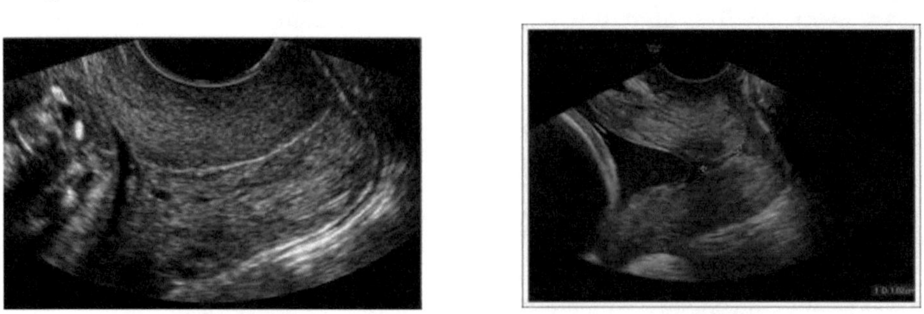

Figure 15.
Transvaginal cervical length measurement showing (a) normal cervix (3.8 cm) and (b) short cervix (1.6 cm).

hence levels >50 ng/mL at >22 weeks gestation is associated with an increased risk of SPTB [92]. However, one should keep in mind that false positive test results can be noted in sexual intercourse, vaginal bleeding, and vaginal lubrication or douching [93].

A qualitative assay involves doing a swab test that detects whether fetal fibronectin is present in the cervicovaginal secretion. A positive fFN test (≥50 ng/mL) has low sensitivity and a positive predictive value [94]. However, a negative fFN test has a high negative predictive value up to 35 weeks gestation and strongly suggests that SPTB will not occur within the following 2 weeks [95]. Due to its limited predictive ability, the American College of Obstetricians and Gynecologists (ACOG) discourages the use of this test as a screening strategy in asymptomatic women, as there is a lack of evidence for better perinatal outcomes.

Quantitative assays are tests that will measure the amount of fetal fibronectin in the cervicovaginal secretions and studies have demonstrated that increasing concentration of qfFN is directly proportional to the rate of SPTB. A threshold of 10 ng/ml has high sensitivity (96%) and negative predictive value (98%) to detect those women unlikely to deliver preterm. The higher the qfFN concentration, the greater the need for surveillance and intervention. It is predicted that quantitative fetal fibronectin measurements enhance the accuracy in the identification of women at risk of preterm delivery [87]. However, studies have shown that combined fFN assay and cervical length screening had low sensitivity to predict SPTB before 35 weeks gestation which was ratified in a systematic review by Berghella et al. [91].

3.3.4 Role of Insulin-like growth factor binding protein (IGFBP-1)

Insulin-like growth factor binding protein-1 (IGFBP-1) is one of the major secretory proteins of the decidualized endometrium and is present in large amounts in the amniotic fluid. Decidua contains more phosphorylated IGFBP-1 (phIGFBP-1) and amniotic fluid contains more nonphosphorylated IGFBP-1. So, when there is a detachment of the fetal membrane, phIGFBP-1 may leak into cervical secretions and trigger the cascade of SPTB. A strong phIGFBP-1-positive result which is an immunochromatography-based dipstick test predicted delivery before 35 completed weeks with a sensitivity of 72.7%, a specificity of 83%, a PPV of 47%, and a negative predictive value of 93.6% [96]. The advantage of this test over fFN is that IGFBP-1 is less prone to influence by sexual intercourse [97].

3.3.5 Role of placental alpha microglobulin 1 (PAMG-1)

PAMG-1 is another glycoprotein synthesized by the decidua and is present in the amniotic fluid in high concentrations. There is a transudation of PAMG-1 through chorioamniotic pores in fetal membranes during uterine contractions due to the inflammatory process of labor or infection. An immunoassay bedside 'dipstick test' is done by a vaginal swab between 20 and 37 weeks to obtain the result within 5 min. This test has a high specificity of 97.5% and NPV of 97.5% and the advantage is that the test results will not be affected by vaginal examination, and thus can be used shortly after the vaginal examination [98].

3.3.6 Role of biomarkers

Certain pro-inflammatory cytokines, such as interleukins, tumor necrosis factor-alpha (TNF-α), C-reactive protein (CRP), granulocyte colony-stimulating factor (G-

CSF), soluble intercellular adhesion molecule-1 (sICAM-1), alkaline phosphatase, stromal cell-derived factor-1a (SDF-1a), interferon-c, and matrix metalloproteinase-8 (MMP-8) are hypothesized to respond to infection at the maternal-fetal interface and stimulate the release of prostaglandins thereby causing uterine contractility and subsequent cervical change triggering SPTB. Based on this concept, an assay of these biomarkers should predict spontaneous preterm birth in women with singleton pregnancies with no symptoms of preterm labor [99]. However, multiple studies and a subsequent meta-analysis by Agudelo et al. have proven that none of the novel biomarkers are clinically useful for predicting SPTB [95, 98] and more research is needed to clarify their efficacy as predictors.

3.3.7 Preventive strategies for SPTB

a. Though OPPTIMUM trial which was designed to determine the role of progesterone in preventing SPTB concluded that progesterone supplementation did not reduce the incidence of preterm birth [100], a subsequent systematic review of randomized controlled trials has proven that vaginal progesterone supplementation starting in the mid trimester to 37 weeks gestation remains the best-known strategy to prevent SPTB in women with a history of prior PTB [101–109]. In addition, vaginal progesterone administration was associated with a reduction in the risk of admission to the neonatal intensive care unit (NICU), respiratory distress syndrome (RDS), composite neonatal morbidity and mortality, and birthweight <1500 g. Vaginal progesterone has been recommended for patients with a singleton gestation and a short cervix by the Society for Maternal-Fetal Medicine (SMFM), the American College of Obstetricians and Gynecologists (ACOG), the International Federation of Gynecology and Obstetrics (FIGO), and the National Institute for Health and Care Excellence (NICE) [110–113].

b. Cervical cerclage, a stitch inserted into the cervix, introduced way back in 1902, is still considered one of the standard options for prophylactic intervention to prevent preterm birth and second trimester fetal loss. Revised nomenclature has been proposed by the NICE in their recent guideline based on the indication of cervical cerclage [114, 115].

A. **History indicated**—a cervical suture which is performed as a prophylactic measure in asymptomatic women but with a history of three or more preterm births or mid trimester losses, is usually inserted as a planned procedure at 11–14 weeks of gestation.

B. **USG indicated**—women with a previous history of one or more spontaneous preterm births or mid trimester losses who are undergoing ultrasound surveillance of cervical length should be offered cerclage if the cervical length is <25 mm < 24 weeks.

C. **Emergency cerclage** (rescue cerclage)—insertion of cerclage as a salvage measure in the case of premature cervical dilatation with exposed fetal membranes in the vagina identified by a speculum or USG can be performed up to 28 weeks.

The different types of cervical stitch are McDonald cerclage which involves placing a transvaginal purse-string suture at the cervical isthmus junction, without bladder mobilization [116]. High transvaginal or Shirodkar cerclage involves placing a transvaginal purse-string suture above the level of the cardinal ligaments following bladder mobilization, [117] and transabdominal cerclage which involves placing the suture at the cervicoisthmic junction by laparotomy or laparoscopy [118]. Transabdominal cerclage can be performed in women with previous unsuccessful transvaginal cerclage and is done in the preconception period or early pregnancy.

3.4 Screening for diabetes

Screening and prediction of diabetes in pregnancy are advisable as it causes increased morbidity, namely fetal macrosomia, trauma during birth, induction of labor, increased chance of cesarean section, shoulder dystocia, neonatal hypoglycemia, and perinatal death. Early diagnosis will ensure the patient follows medical nutritional therapy along with exercise and if glycemic control is not achieved, early recourse to oral hypoglycemic agents or Insulin can be undertaken thereby preventing the abovementioned morbidity.

The risk factors for the development of diabetes in pregnancy are:

- BMI above 30 kg/m^2
- previous macrosomic baby weighing 4.5 kg or above
- previous h/o gestational diabetes
- family history of diabetes
- ethnicity with a high prevalence of diabetes

Screening is done by the 75-g 2-h oral glucose tolerance test (OGTT) to test for gestational diabetes in women with risk factors. Women who had gestational diabetes in a previous pregnancy, can either be offered early self-monitoring of blood glucose or a 75-g 2-h OGTT as soon as possible after booking (whether in the first or second trimester) and a further 75-g 2-h OGTT at 24–28 weeks if the results of the first OGTT are normal. In women with no risk factors, OGTT is offered at 24–28 weeks. Gestational diabetes mellitus (GDM) is diagnosed if the fasting plasma glucose level is 5.6 mmol/L or above or a 2-h plasma glucose level is 7.8 mmol/L or above and the woman is advised a dietician consultation and medical nutrition therapy (MNT-Diet/exercise) is initiated. If her glycemic control is inadequate within 2 weeks, she should be referred to a diabetologist for the start of oral hypoglycemic agents (OHA)/Insulin. In a woman with preexisting DM, multidisciplinary team care should be offered for optimal glycemic control and adequate end-organ assessment from preconception to delivery [119].

3.5 USG to screen for anomalies

USG has been established as an essential modality in the prenatal assessment of the fetus and thus obtain an optimal outcome for the mother and fetus. As a majority of fetal abnormalities occur in the low-risk group, targeted imaging of fetal anomalies is offered to all pregnant women. The mid trimester USG is done between 18 and

24 weeks of gestation according to the local protocol regarding the legal limit of termination of pregnancy. The sensitivity in detecting anomalies improves when done in close to 24 weeks. The request for the scan should originate from the primary obstetrician and the pregnant woman should be counseled regarding the potential benefits and limitations of a second trimester fetal ultrasound scan and a consent form should be signed before the evaluation. Mid trimester USG should be performed by trained professionals, and it includes a detailed and systematic evaluation of the external and internal anatomy of the fetus. The established accuracy in diagnosing fetal anomalies according to the EUROFETUS study is 55–60% [120].

For the mid trimester scans, a USG machine with the following capabilities should be used: real-time, grayscale transabdominal/transvaginal transducers, necessary software applications, color Doppler, power Doppler, adjustable acoustic power output controls with output display standards, freeze-frame capabilities, electronic calipers, and capacity to print/store images. High-end machines with elaborate software settings and the use of 3D/4D probes will hasten the diagnosis and reporting process in certain circumstances.

Though the safety of USG has been established in many studies [121–123], the evaluation time should be minimized, using the lowest possible power output needed to obtain diagnostic information, following the as low as reasonably achievable (ALARA) principle [124]. Apart from evaluation of cardiac activity, fetal number, fetal environment, placental appearance and location, evaluation of biometry to assess fetal growth is recommended in the mid trimester USG. Biometry includes biparietal diameter (BPD), head circumference (HC), abdominal circumference (AC), and femur length (FL). Details of evaluation and images of mandatory biometry are given in **Table 8**. The minimum evaluation and checklist which is recommended in the mid trimester USG are described in **Table 9** [125].

Biometry	Plane studied	USG image
BPD, HC	Transthalamic	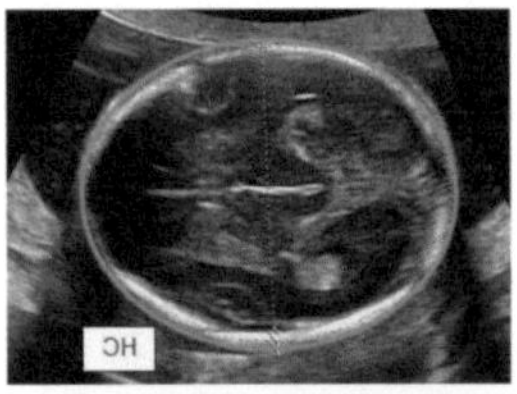
AC	Axial section of abdomen at the level of stomach bubble, confluence of the umbilical vein and portal sinus	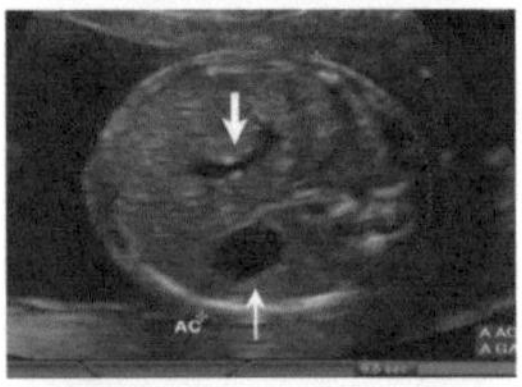
FL	Distance between the two metaphyses with an angle <45°	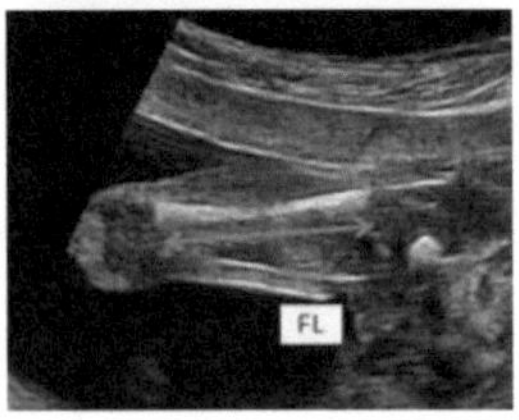

Table 8.
Planes of evaluation and images of mandatory biometry in mid trimester scan.

Anatomic region	Structures assessed
Head	Intact skull, midline falx, cavum septi pellucidi, cerebral lateral ventricles, thalami, cerebellum, cisterna magna
Face	Both orbits, midsagittal facial profile, nose and mouth with an intact upper lip
Neck	Absence of cysts and masses
Spine	Sagittal, coronal, and axial views showing no open neural tube defects
Thorax	Normal shape/size of chest and lungs Cardiac situs, Four-chamber view of heart, Aortic and pulmonary outflow tracts No evidence of diaphragmatic hernia
Abdomen	Stomach in normal position, bowel not dilated, both kidneys present, Cord insertion site-normal
Extremities	Three segments of all four limbs with normal relationship, arms and feet present, normal muscle mass
Placenta	Position, no masses present, any accessory lobe
Umbilical cord	Three vessel cord

Table 9.
Minimum requirements recommended in 18–24 weeks USG (modified from ISUOG practice guideline for mid-trimester USG, 2011).

Evaluation of the cervix, uterine pathology like fibroids and adnexa also should be done to look for any pathology. A proper referral mechanism should be in place once a diagnosis of an anomaly is made and a detailed report including the name, date of USG, any relevant medical or obstetric conditions, the scan indication, the best estimate of gestational age, estimated delivery date, amniotic fluid assessment, BPD, HC, AC, and FL (in centiles), EFW in grams with centile graphs, Dopplers, diagnostic impression, and recommendations for follow up examination or management.

Thus, the inverted care pyramid model helps in the identification of low, intermediate, and high-risk antenatal mothers. The low-risk mothers continue their antenatal care in the general obstetrician's clinic, the high-risk group is treated by a multidisciplinary team including perinatologists, genetic counselors, dieticians, endocrinologists, and USG experts. The intermediate group in their further visits is stratified as either high or low-risk groups and managed accordingly.

4. Postnatal period

Care during this period is based on the concept that the prevalence of various NCD, namely metabolic syndromes and premature cardiovascular diseases is increased in women with uteroplacental dysfunction. These women are referred to specialist care, namely diabetologists, nephrologists, endocrinologists, genetic counselors, cardiologists, and nutritionists thereby preventing future occurrence of NCDs. This can be achieved using lifestyle changes, exercise, and medication. Furthermore, the women who have preexisting medical morbidities like connective tissue disorders, renal disease, and neurological disease are referred to appropriate specialist physicians for a reevaluation of their medical condition and alteration of medication if indicated.

5. Conclusion

Incorporation of the above-mentioned protocols in the prenatal screening process helps in the standardization of antenatal care from the preconception period, into the pregnancy till delivery, and through the postnatal period. This structured care will help in the substantial reduction of adverse outcomes in pregnancy thus achieving an optimal perinatal outcome. Thus, prenatal screening helps us to predict the at-risk mother and fetus, and prevent the problem from occurring by means of prophylactic measures and timely interventions. Nevertheless, in unpreventable conditions, a multidisciplinary team-based approach is considered and relevant care is given to both mother and fetus to make the process of delivery and the postnatal period a less stressful and more pleasant one.

Acknowledgement

This chapter is dedicated to "Roshan Jethro Rollands, my son, my guardian angel."

Author details

Brinda Sabu* and Vidyalekshmy Ranganayaki
Department of High-Risk Pregnancy and Perinatology, KIMSHEALTH, Trivandrum, Kerala, India

*Address all correspondence to: brinda_sabu@yahoo.co.in

References

[1] WHO, UNICEF, UNFPA, World Bank Group, and the United Nations Population Division. Maternal Mortality: Levels and Trends 2000 to 2017. Geneva: 2019. Available from: https://www.who.int/reproductivehealth/publications/maternalmortality-2000-2017/

[2] Ministry of Health Report. 1929. Memorandum on Antenatal Clinics: Their Conduct and Scope. London: His Majesty's Stationery Office; 1930

[3] Nicolaides KH. Turning the pyramid of prenatal care. Fetal Diagnosis and Therapy. 2011;**29**:184

[4] Hod M, Kypros N. Merging the legacies and hypotheses—Maternal medicine meets fetal medicine. In: Textbook of DM in Pregnancy. 3rd ed. Florida: CRC Press, Taylor and Francis Group; 2016. pp. 1-8

[5] Nicolaides K. A model for a new pyramid of prenatal care based on the 11 to 13 weeks' assessment. Prenatal Diagnosis. 2011;**31**:3-6

[6] Ljubić A. Inverted pyramid of prenatal care—Is it enough? Should it be—Extended inverted pyramid of prenatal care? Journal of Perinatal Medicine. Sep 25, 2018;**46**(7):716-720. DOI: 10.1515/jpm-2016-0427. PMID: 28593902

[7] Urato AC, Norwitz ER. A guide towards pre-pregnancy management of defective implantation and placentation. Best Practice & Research. Clinical Obstetrics & Gynaecology. 2011;**25**: 367-387

[8] Cell-free DNA screening for fetal aneuploidy. Committee Opinion No. 640. American College of Obstetricians and Gynecologists. Obstetrics and Gynecology. 2015;**126**:31-37

[9] Society for Maternal-Fetal Medicine (SMFM) Publications Committee. #36: Prenatal aneuploidy screening using cell-free DNA. American Journal of Obstetrics and Gynecology. 2015;**212**: 711-716

[10] Wald NJ, Rodeck C, Hackshaw AK, Walkers J, Chitty L, Mackinson AM, et al. First and second-trimester antenatal screening for Down's syndrome: The results of the serum, urine, and ultrasound screening study (SURUSS). Health Technology Assessment. 2003;**7**:1-77

[11] Exalto N, Steegers EA. Robinson's crown-rump length curve—A major step towards human embryonic health evaluation. BJOG: International Journal of Obstetrics and Gynaecology. 2018; **126**(3):310

[12] Napolitano R, Dhami J, Ohuma EO, Ioannou C, Conde-Agudelo A, Kennedy SH, et al. Pregnancy dating by fetal crown-rump length: A systematic review of charts. BJOG. Apr 2014; **121**(5):556-565. DOI: 10.1111/1471-0528.12478. Epub 2014 Jan 6. PMID: 24387345

[13] Folsom AR, Shah AM, Lutsey PL, et al. American Heart Association's Life's simple 7: Avoiding heart failure and preserving cardiac structure and function. American Journal of Medicine. 2015;**128**:970-976

[14] Loane M, Morris JK, Addor M, Arriola L, Budd J, Doray B, et al. Twenty-year trends in the prevalence of Down syndrome and other trisomies in Europe: Impact of maternal age and

prenatal screening. European Journal of Human Genetics. 2013;**21**:27-33

[15] Parker SE, Mai CT, Canfield MA, Rickard R, Wang Y, Meyer RE, et al. Updated national birth prevalence estimates for selected birth defects in the United States, 2004–2006. Birth Defects Research. Part A, Clinical and Molecular Teratology. 2010;**88**:1008-1016

[16] Morin L, Lim K. SOGC Diagnostic Imaging Committee; SOGC Genetics Committee; SOGC Maternal-Fetal Medicine Committee. Ultrasound for twin pregnancies. SOGC Clinical Practice Guideline No. 260, June 2011. Journal of Obstetrics and Gynaecology Canada. 2011;**33**:643-656

[17] Machin GA. Why is it important to diagnose chorionicity and how do we do it? Best Practice & Research. Clinical Obstetrics & Gynaecology. 2004;**18**: 515-530

[18] Sepulveda W, Sebire NJ, Hughes K, et al. The lambda sign at 10-14 weeks of gestation as a predictor of chorionicity in twin pregnancies. Ultrasound in Obstetrics & Gynecology. 1996;**7**:421-423

[19] Shetty A, Smith AP. The sonographic diagnosis of chorionicity. Prenatal Diagnosis. 2005;**25**:735-739

[20] Dube J, Dodds L, Armson BA. Does chorionicity or zygosity predict adverse perinatal outcomes in twins? American Journal of Obstetrics and Gynecology. 2002;**186**:579-583

[21] Sebire NJ, Snijders RJ, Hughes K, et al. The hidden mortality of monochorionic twin pregnancies. British Journal of Obstetrics and Gynaecology. 1997;**104**:1203-1207

[22] Nicolaides KH, Azar G, Byrne D, Mansur C, Marks K. Fetal nuchal translucency: Ultrasound screening for fetal trisomy in the first trimester of pregnancy. BMJ. 1992;**304**: 867-869

[23] Ville Y, Lalondrelle C, Doumerc S, Daffos F, Frydman R, Oury JF, et al. First-trimester diagnosis of nuchal anomalies: Significance and fetal outcome. Ultrasound in Obstetrics & Gynecology. 1992;**2**:314-316

[24] American Institute of Ultrasound in Medicine (AIUM). AIUM practice guideline for the performance of obstetric ultrasound examinations. Journal of Ultrasound in Medicine. 2013; **32**:1083-1101

[25] Hui L, Pynaker C, Bonacquisto L, et al. Re-examining the optimal nuchal translucency cutoff for diagnostic testing in the cell-free DNA and microarray era: Results from the Victorian perinatal record linkage study. American Journal of Obstetrics and Gynecology. 2021;**225** (5):527.e1-527.e12

[26] Nicolaides KH. The 11–13+6 Weeks Scan. London: Fetal Medicine Foundation; 2004

[27] Spencer K, Liao A, Skentou H, Cicero S, Nicolaides K. Screening for Triploidy by Fetal nuchal translucency and maternal serum free B-hCG and PAPP-A at 10-14 weeks of gestation. Prenatal Diagnosis. 2000;**20**(6): 495-499

[28] Bush MC, Malone FD. Down syndrome screening in twins. Clinics in Perinatology. 2005;**32**:373-386

[29] Dashe JS. Aneuploidy screening in pregnancy. Obstetrics & Gynecology. 2016;**128**(1):181-194. DOI: 10.1097/AOG.0000000 000001385

[30] Baer RJ, Flessel MC, Jellife-Pawlowski LL, Goldman S, Hudgins L, Hull AD, et al. Detection rates for aneuploidy by first-trimester and sequential screening. Obstetrics and Gynecology. 2015;**126**:753-759

[31] Gil MM, Quezada MS, Revello R, Akolekar R, Nicolaides KH. Analysis of cell-free DNA in maternal blood in screening for fetal aneuploidies: An updated meta-analysis. Ultrasound in Obstetrics & Gynecology. 2015;**45**: 249-266

[32] Norton ME, Jacobsson B, Swamy GK, Laurent LC, Ranzini AC, Brar H, et al. Cell-free DNA analysis for noninvasive examination of trisomy. The New England Journal of Medicine. 2015; **372**:1589-1597

[33] Cuckle HS, Malone FD, Wright D, Porter TF, Nyberg DA, Comstock CH, et al. Contingent screening for Down syndrome- results from the FaSTER trial. Prenatal Diagnosis. 2008;**28**:89-94

[34] Zhang H, Gao Y, Jiang F, Fu M, Yuan Y, Guo Y, et al. Noninvasive prenatal testing for trisomies 21, 18, and 13: Clinical experience from 146,958 pregnancies. Ultrasound in Obstetrics & Gynecology. 2015;**45**:530-538

[35] Pergament E, Cuckle H, Zimmermann B, Banjevic M, Sigurjonsson S, Ryan A, et al. Single-nucleotide polymorphism based noninvasive prenatal screening in a high-risk and low-risk cohort. Obstetrics and Gynecology. 2014;**124**:210-218

[36] Curnow KJ, Wilkins-Haug L, Ryan A, Kirkizlar E, Stosic M, Hall MP, et al. Detection of triploid, molar, and vanishing twin pregnancies by single-nucleotide polymorphism-based noninvasive prenatal test. American Journal of Obstetrics and Gynecology. 2015;**212**(79):e1-e9

[37] Grati FR, Malvestiti F, Ferreira JC, Bajaj K, Gaetani E, Agrati C, et al. Fetoplacental mosaicism: Potential implications for false-positive and false-negative non-invasive prenatal screening results. Genetics in Medicine. 2014;**16**: 620-624

[38] Bianchi DW, Chudova D, Sehnert AJ, Bhatt S, Murray K, Prosen TL, et al. Non-invasive prenatal testing and incidental detection of occult maternal malignancies. JAMA. 2015;**314**:162-169

[39] Wang Y, Chen Y, Tian F, Zhang J, Song Z, Wu Y, et al. Maternal mosaicism is a significant contributor to discordant sex chromosomal aneuploidies associated with non-invasive prenatal testing. Clinical Chemistry. 2014;**60**:251-259

[40] Bianchi DW, Parker RL, Wentworth J, Madankumar R, Saffer C, Das AF, et al. DNA sequencing versus standard prenatal aneuploidy screening. The New England Journal of Medicine. 2014;**370**: 799-808

[41] Dar P, Curnow KJ, Gross SJ, Hall MP, Stosic M, Demko Z, et al. Clinical experience and follow-up with large scale single-nucleotide polymorphism-based noninvasive prenatal aneuploidy testing. American Journal of Obstetrics and Gynecology. 2014;**211**(527):e1-e17

[42] Brar H, Wang E, Struble C, Musci TJ, Norton ME. The fetal fraction of cell-free DNA in maternal plasma is not affected by a priori risk of fetal trisomy. The Journal of Maternal-Fetal & Neonatal Medicine. 2013;**26**:143-145

[43] Quezada MS, Gil MM, Francisco C, Orosz G, Nicolaides KH. Screening for trisomies 21, 18, and 13 by cell-free DNA

analysis of maternal blood at 10–11 weeks' gestation and the combined test at 11–13 weeks. Ultrasound in Obstetrics & Gynecology. 2015;**45**:36-41

[44] Norton ME, Jelliffe-Pawlowski LL, Currier RJ. Chromosome abnormalities are detected by current prenatal screening and noninvasive prenatal testing. Obstetrics and Gynecology. 2014;**124**:979-986

[45] American College of Obstetricians and Gynecologists. Screening for fetal aneuploidy. Practice Bulletin No. 163. Obstetrics and Gynecology. 2016;**127**: 123-137

[46] Vintzileos AM, Egan JF. Adjusting the risk for trisomy 21 based on second-trimester ultrasonography. American Journal of Obstetrics and Gynecology. 1995;**172**:837-844

[47] Kim MS, Kang S, Cho HY. Clinical significance of sonographic soft markers: A review. Journal of Genetic Medicine. 2018;**15**:1-7

[48] Agathokleous M, Chaveeva P, Poon LC, Kosinski P, Nicolaides KH. Meta-analysis of second-trimester markers for trisomy 21. Ultrasound in Obstetrics & Gynecology. 2013;**41**:247-261

[49] Baffero GM, Somigliana E, Crovetto F, et al. Confined placental mosaicism at chorionic villous sampling: Risk factors and pregnancy outcome. Prenatal Diagnosis. 2012;**32**(11):1102-1108

[50] Akolekar R, Beta J, Picciarelli G, et al. Procedure-related risk of miscarriage following amniocentesis and chorionic villus sampling: A systematic review and meta-analysis. Ultrasound in Obstetrics & Gynecology. 2015;**45**(1):16-26

[51] Practice bulletin No. 162: Prenatal diagnostic testing for genetic disorders. Obstetrics and Gynecology. 2016;**127**(5): 108-122

[52] Audibert F, Wilson RD, Allen V, et al. Preimplantation genetic testing. Journal of Obstetrics and Gynaecology Canada. 2009;**31**(8):761-775

[53] DeUgarte CM, Li M, Surrey M, et al. Accuracy of FISH analysis in predicting chromosomal status in patients undergoing preimplantation genetic diagnosis. Fertility and Sterility. 2008;**90** (4):1049-1054

[54] Leona P, Syngelaki A, Akolekar R, Nicolaides K. Combined screening for preeclampsia and small for gestational age at 11–13 weeks. Fetal Diagnosis and Therapy. 2013;**33**:16-27

[55] Tranquilli AL, Dekker G, Magee L, et al. The classification, diagnosis, and management of the hypertensive disorders of pregnancy: A revised statement from the ISSHP. Pregnancy Hypertens. 2014;**4**:97-104

[56] Magee LA, Pels A, Helewa M, Rey E, von Dadelszen P, Canadian Hypertensive Disorders of Pregnancy (HDP) Working Group. Diagnosis, evaluation, and management of the hypertensive disorders of pregnancy. Pregnancy Hypertens. 2014;**4**:105-145

[57] Villar J, Say L, Gulmezoglu AM, et al. Eclampsia and pre-eclampsia: A health problem for 2000 years. In: Critchly H, MacLean A, Post L, Walk J, editors. Pre-Eclampsia. London: RCOG Press; 2003. pp. 189-207

[58] Ronsmans C, Graham WJ. Maternal mortality: Who, when, where, and why. Lancet. 2006;**368**:1189-1200

[59] Brown MA, Magee LA, Kenny LC, et al. The hypertensive disorders of pregnancy: ISSHP classification,

diagnosis & management recommendations for international practice. Pregnancy Hypertens. 2018;**13**: 291-310

[60] Beck DW, Menezes AH. Intracerebral hemorrhage in a patient with eclampsia. Journal of the American Medical Association. 1981;**246**: 1442-1443

[61] Zhang J, Meikle S, Trumble A. Severe maternal morbidity associated with hypertensive disorders in pregnancy in the United States. Hypertension in Pregnancy. 2003;**22**: 203-212

[62] National Collaborating Centre for women's and Children's Health (UK). In: Hypertension in Pregnancy: The Management of Hypertensive Disorders during Pregnancy. London: RCOG Press; 2010

[63] Poon LC, Zymeri NA, Zamprakou A, Syngelaki A, Nicolaides KH. Protocol for measurement of mean arterial pressure at 11-13 weeks' gestation. Fetal Diagnosis and Therapy. 2012;**31**:42-48

[64] Poon LC, Shennan A, Romero R, Nicolaides KH, Hod M. The International Federation of Gynecology and Obstetrics (FIGO) initiative on pre-eclampsia: A pragmatic guide for first-trimester screening and prevention. International Journal of Gynecology & Obstetrics. 2019;**145**(Suppl. 1):1-33

[65] Sotiriadis A, Hernandez-Andrade E, da Silva CF, et al. ISUOG practice guidelines: Role of ultrasound in screening for and follow-up of pre-eclampsia. Ultrasound in Obstetrics & Gynecology. 2019;**53**:7-22

[66] Levine RJ, Maynard SE, Qian C, et al. Circulating angiogenic factors and the risk of preeclampsia. The New England Journal of Medicine. 2004;**350**: 672-683

[67] Ahmad S, Ahmed A. Elevated placental soluble vascular endothelial growth factor receptor-1 inhibits angiogenesis in preeclampsia. Circulation Research. 2004;**95**:884-891

[68] Chau K, Hennessy A, Makris A. Placental growth factor and preeclampsia. Journal of Human Hypertension. 2017;**31**:782-786

[69] Wortelboer EJ, Koster MP, Kuc S, et al. Longitudinal trends in fetoplacental biochemical markers, uterine artery pulsatility index and maternal blood pressure during the first trimester of pregnancy. Ultrasound in Obstetrics & Gynecology. 2011;**38**:383-388

[70] Tidwell SC, Ho HN, Chiu WH, Torry RJ, Torry DS. Low maternal serum levels of placenta growth factor as an antecedent of clinical preeclampsia. American Journal of Obstetrics and Gynecology. 2001;**184**:1267-1272

[71] Thadhani R, Mutter WP, Wolf M, et al. First-trimester placental growth factor and soluble fms-like tyrosine kinase 1 and risk for preeclampsia. The Journal of Clinical Endocrinology and Metabolism. 2004;**89**:770-775

[72] Rolnik DL, Wright D, Poon LCY, Syngelaki A, O'Gorman N, de Paco Matallana C, et al. ASPRE trial: Performance of screening for preterm pre-eclampsia. Ultrasound in Obstetrics & Gynecology. 2017;**50**:492-495

[73] Verlohren S, Herraiz I, Lapaire O, Schlembach D, Moertl M, Zeisler H, et al. The sFlt-1/PlGF ratio in different types of hypertensive pregnancy disorders and its prognostic potential in

preeclamptic patients. American Journal of Obstetrics and Gynecology. 2012;**206** (58):1-8

[74] Zeisler H, Llurba E, Chantraine F, Vatish M, Staff AC, Sennstrom M, et al. Soluble fms-like tyrosine kinase-1-to-placental growth factor ratio and time to delivery in women with suspected preeclampsia. Obstetrics and Gynecology. 2016;**128**:261-269

[75] Villa PM, Hamalainen E, Maki A, Raikkonen K, Pesonen AK, Taipale P, et al. Vasoactive agents for the prediction of early- and late-onset preeclampsia in a high-risk cohort. BMC Pregnancy and Childbirth. 2013;**13**:110

[76] Zeisler H, Llurba E, Chantraine F, Vatish M, Staff AC, Sennstrom M, et al. Predictive value of the sFlt-1:PlGF ratio in women with suspected preeclampsia. The New England Journal of Medicine. 2016;**374**:13-22

[77] Bian X, Biswas A, Huang X, Lee KJ, Li TK, Masuyama H, et al. Short-term prediction of adverse outcomes using the sFlt-1 (soluble fms-like tyrosine kinase 1)/PlGF (placental growth factor) ratio in Asian women with suspected preeclampsia. Hypertension. 2019;**74**: 164-172

[78] Magee LA, Dadelszen PV, Stones WM. The FIGO Textbook of Pregnancy Hypertension. An Evidence-Based Guide to Monitoring, Prevention, and Management. London: The Global Library of Woman's Medicine; 2016

[79] Morisaki N, Togoobaatar G, Vogel JP, et al. Risk factors for spontaneous and provider-initiated preterm delivery in high and low human development index countries: A secondary analysis of the World Health Organization Multicountry Survey on Maternal and Newborn Health. Journal of Obstetrics and Gynaecology. 2014;**121**(Suppl. 1): 101-109

[80] Platt MJ. Outcomes in preterm infants. Public Health. 2014;**128**:399-403

[81] Howson CP, Kinney MV, McDougall L, Lawn JE. Born too soon: Preterm birth matters. Reproductive Health. 2013;**10** (Suppl. 1):S1

[82] Goldenberg RL, Culhane JF, Iams JD, Romero R. Epidemiology and causes of preterm birth. Lancet. 2008;**371**:75-84

[83] American College of Obstetricians and Gynecologists. Practice bulletin No. 171: Management of preterm labor. Obstetrics and Gynecology. 2016;**128**: 155-164

[84] Marlow N, Wolke D, Bracewell MA, Samara M. Neurologic and developmental disability at six years of age after extremely preterm birth. The New England Journal of Medicine. 2005; **352**:9-19

[85] Culhane JF, Goldenberg RL. Racial disparities in preterm birth. Seminars in Perinatology. 2011;**35**:234-239

[86] Goldenberg RL, Iams JD, Mercer BM, et al. What we have learned about the predictors of preterm birth. Seminars in Perinatology. 2003;**27**:185-193

[87] Abbott DS, Hezelgrave NL, Seed PT, et al. Quantitative fetal fibronectin to predict preterm birth in asymptomatic women at high risk. Obstetrics and Gynecology. 2015;**125**:1168-1176

[88] Esplin MS, Elovitz MA, Iams JD, et al. Predictive accuracy of serial transvaginal cervical lengths and quantitative vaginal fetal fibronectin levels for spontaneous preterm birth among nulliparous women. JAMA. 2017; **317**:1047-1056

[89] Owen J, Yost N, Berghella V, et al. Mid-trimester endovaginal sonography in women at high risk for spontaneous preterm birth. JAMA. 2001;**286**: 1340-1348

[90] Jwala S, Tran TL, Terenna C, et al. Evaluation of additive effect of quantitative fetal fibronectin to cervical length for prediction of spontaneous preterm birth among asymptomatic low-risk women. Acta Obstetricia et Gynecologica Scandinavica. 2016;**95**: 948-955

[91] Berghella V, Hayes E, Visintine J, Baxter JK. Fetal fibronectin testing for reducing the risk of preterm birth. Cochrane Database of Systematic Reviews. 2008;(4):CD006843

[92] Bastek JA, Elovitz MA. The role and challenges of biomarkers in spontaneous preterm birth and preeclampsia. Fertility and Sterility. 2013;**99**:1117-1123

[93] Wei SQ, Fraser W, Luo ZC. Inflammatory cytokines and spontaneous preterm birth in asymptomatic women: A systematic review. Obstetrics and Gynecology. 2010;**116**:393-401

[94] Lucaroni F, Morciano L, Rizzo G, D' Antonio F, Buonuomo E, Palombi L, et al. Biomarkers for predicting spontaneous preterm birth: An umbrella systematic review. The Journal of Maternal-Fetal & Neonatal Medicine. Mar 2018;**31**(6):726-734. DOI: 10.1080/14767058.2017.1297404. Epub 2017 Mar 8. PMID: 28274163

[95] Conde-Agudelo A, Papageorghiou AT, Kennedy SH, Villar J. Novel biomarkers for the prediction of the spontaneous preterm birth phenotype: A systematic review and meta-analysis. British Journal of Obstetrics and Gynaecology. 2011;**118**:1042-1054

[96] Conde-Agudelo A, RomeroR. Cervical phosphorylated insulin-like growth factor binding protein-1 test for the prediction of preterm birth: A systematic review and meta-analysis. American Journal of Obstetrics and Gynecology. 2016;**214**(1): 57-73

[97] McLaren JS, Hezelgrave NL, Ayubi H, Seed PT, Shennan AH. Prediction of spontaneous preterm birth using quantitative fetal fibronectin after recent sexual intercourse. American Journal of Obstetrics and Gynecology. 2015;**212**(1): 89.1-89.5

[98] Goldenberg RL, Goepfert AR, Ramsey PS. Biochemical markers for the prediction of preterm birth. American Journal of Obstetrics and Gynecology. 2005;**5**(Suppl):S36-S46

[99] Glover AV, Manuck TA. Screening for spontaneous preterm birth and resultant therapies to reduce neonatal morbidity and mortality: A review. Seminars in Fetal & Neonatal Medicine. 2018;**23**(2):126-132. DOI: 10.1016/j.siny.2017.11.007

[100] Norman JE, Marlow N, Messow CM, et al. Vaginal progesterone prophylaxis for preterm birth (the OPPTIMUM study): A multicentre, randomized, double-blind trial. Lancet. 2016;**387**:2106-2116

[101] Khalifeh A, Berghella V. Universal cervical length screening in singleton gestations without a previous preterm birth: Ten reasons why it should be implemented. American Journal of Obstetrics and Gynecology. 2016;**214**: 603.1-603.5

[102] Romero R, Yeo L, Chaemsaithong P, Chaiworapongsa T, Hassan SS. Progesterone to prevent spontaneous

preterm birth. Seminars in Fetal & Neonatal Medicine. 2014;**19**:15-26

[103] Campbell S. Universal cervical-length screening and vaginal progesterone prevents early preterm births, reduces neonatal morbidity, and is cost-saving: Doing nothing is no longer an option. Ultrasound in Obstetrics & Gynecology. 2011;**38**:1-9

[104] Iams JD. Clinical practice. Prevention of preterm parturition. The New England Journal of Medicine. 2014; **370**:254-261

[105] Conde-Agudelo A, Romero R. Vaginal progesterone to prevent preterm birth in pregnant women with a sonographic short cervix: Clinical and public health implications. American Journal of Obstetrics and Gynecology. 2016;**214**:235-242

[106] O'brien JM, Lewis DF. Prevention of preterm birth with vaginal progesterone or 17-alpha hydroxyprogesterone caproate: A critical examination of efficacy and safety. American Journal of Obstetrics and Gynecology. 2016;**214**:45-56

[107] Vintzileos AM, Visser GH. Interventions for women with a mid-trimester short cervix: Which ones work? Ultrasound in Obstetrics & Gynecology. 2017;**49**:295-300

[108] Pedretti MK, Kazemier BM, Dickinson JE, Mol BW. Implementing universal cervical length screening in asymptomatic women with singleton pregnancies: Challenges and opportunities. The Australian & New Zealand Journal of Obstetrics & Gynaecology. 2017;**57**:221-227

[109] Romero R, Fonseca E, O'Brien J, Nicolaides K. Vaginal progesterone for preventing preterm birth and adverse perinatal outcomes in singleton gestations with a short cervix: A meta-analysis of individual patient data. Available from: https://www.sciencedirect.com/science/article/pii/S0002937817323438

[110] Progesterone and preterm birth prevention: Translating clinical trials data into clinical practice. American Journal of Obstetrics and Gynecology. 2012;**206**:376-386

[111] Practice bulletin no. 130: Prediction and prevention of preterm birth. Obstetrics and Gynecology. 2012;**120**: 964-973

[112] Figo Working Group on Best Practice in Maternal-Fetal M. Best practice in maternal-fetal medicine. International Journal of Gynaecology and Obstetrics. 2015;**128**:80-82

[113] National Institute for health and care excellence-preterm labor and birth. NICEguideline. 2015. Available from: https://www.nice.org.uk/guidance/ng25/evidence/resources/fullguideline-2176838029

[114] Shennan AH, Story L. The Royal College of Obstetricians, Gynaecologists. Cervical Cerclage. BJOG. 2022;**129**: 1178-1210. DOI: 10.1111/1471-0528.17003

[115] Alfirevic Z, Stampalija T, Medley N. Cervical stitch (cerclage) for preventing preterm birth in singleton pregnancy. Cochrane Database of Systematic Reviews. 2017;**6**:CD008991

[116] McDonald IA. Suture of the cervix for inevitable miscarriage. The Journal of Obstetrics and Gynaecology of the British Empire. 1957;**64**:346-350

[117] Shirodkar VN. A new method of operative treatment for habitual

abortion in the second trimester of pregnancy. Antiseptic. 1955;**52**:299-300

[118] Benson RC, Durfee RB. Transabdominal cervical uterine cerclage during pregnancy for the treatment of cervical incompetency. Obstetrics and Gynecology. 1965;**25**:145-155

[119] The NICE guideline. Diabetes in pregnancy: Management from preconception to the postnatal period. 2015

[120] Grandjean H, Larroque D, Levi S. The performance of routine ultrasonographic screening of pregnancies in the Eurofetus Study, American Journal of Obstetrics and Gynecology. 1999;**181**:446-454

[121] Nelson TR, Fowlkes JB, Abramowicz JS, Church CC. Ultrasound biosafety considerations for the practicing sonographer and sonologist. Journal of Ultrasound in Medicine. 2009;**28**:139-150

[122] Safety Group of the British Medical Ultrasound Society. Guidelines for the safe use of diagnostic ultrasound equipment. Ultrasound. 2010;**2010**(18): 52-59

[123] Harris GR, Church CC, Dalecki D, et al. Comparison of thermal safety practice guidelines for diagnostic ultrasound exposures. Ultrasound in Medicine & Biology. 2016;**42**:345-357

[124] American Institute of Ultrasound in Medicine. AIUM practice guidelines for the performance of obstetric ultrasound examination. Journal of Ultrasound in Medicine. 2010;**29**:157-166

[125] Salomon LJ, Alfirevic Z, Berghella V, Bilardo C, Hernandez AE, Johnsen SL, et al. Practice guidelines for performance of the routine mid-trimester fetal ultrasound scan. Ultrasound in Obstetrics & Gynecology. 2011;**37**: 116-126

Chapter 11

Common Indications and Techniques in Prenatal MRI

Ryan Holman

Abstract

Fetal and perinatal diagnostic imaging with MRI has evolved and expanded during recent times, allowing more widespread use and availability. Common indications are for neurodevelopmental conditions that are inconclusive with ultrasonography. The modality is pivotal in treatment planning for *in utero* interventions, such as repair of neural tube defects, and for particular obstetrical complications. The technique is also useful for identifying neurological sequelae from conditions like congenital heart defects and maternal viral infections. Many other applications are not indicated for routine use, particularly due to the high cost, but show much promise in research applications. Recently, complications associated with COVID-19 have been an area of interest, with prenatal MRI cohorts and case studies reporting obstetrical complications and neurodevelopmental effects. This review is aimed at highlighting common indications for the use of MRI in maternal-fetal medicine, including the MRI sequences and physics often implemented. Also, an in-depth analysis of the SARS-CoV-2 virus is discussed; in addition to pregnancy-related complications and the role of prenatal MRI in diagnosis and treatment.

Keywords: prenatal MRI, fetal MRI, birth defects, obstetrics, radiology, COVID-19

1. Introduction

Infection, preterm birth, and perinatal complications including asphyxia are among the leading causes of neonatal deaths worldwide [1, 2]. Neonatal and antenatal mortality and morbidity is most often associated with preterm birth that can result in respiratory complications, developmental abnormalities, and high-risk of infections [3, 4]. Infection has been reported in approximately 23% of worldwide neonatal deaths with an estimated 84% of instances being preventable with proper medical treatment [1, 5]. Preterm birth results in the majority of neonatal morbidity and mortality, is the direct cause of approximately 35% of neonatal deaths worldwide, and is the major risk factor for all types of neonatal deaths [1, 3, 4, 6]. Hypoxic birth asphyxia is expected to cause approximately 30% of worldwide neonatal mortality, identified by the inability to perform voluntary breathing at birth, can be observed intrapartum with techniques including Doppler ultrasound and auscultation, and can be diagnosed by an arterial pH in the umbilical cord less than 7.2 [7].

Some of the most common birth defects include congenital heart disease (CHD), down syndrome, and neural tube defects. Congenital cardiac complications are the most common form of congenital abnormalities, with an estimated worldwide prevalence in about 0.8% of all live births, resulting in approximately 1/3 of all congenital abnormalities that cause significant medical and social consequences [8, 9]. Down syndrome is expected in about 1 in 400–1500 births, is the most common chromosomal abnormality, can be diagnosed early in pregnancy with chorionic villus sampling or amniocenteses, and predominately results from trisomy of chromosome 21 [10]. Global neural tube defect prevalence is estimated at 0.05–1% of live births, are characterized by improper closure of the neural tube during fetal development, are commonly asymptomatic, with spina bifida being the most common type, of which the most severe is myelomeningocele [11–13].

The understanding of normal *in utero* fetal brain development is still largely unknown, with techniques like magnetic resonance imaging (MRI) being uncommon in absence of disease [14]. Fetal MRI has allowed better understanding of the physiological processes involved with normal neurodevelopmental maturation, *in utero* and *ex utero* comparison, the underpinnings of congenital disease mechanisms, and long-term outcomes for specific conditions [14–17]. In the clinic, fetal MRI is often undertaken after referral from a maternal-fetal medicine specialist and indicated to help in diagnosis of particular conditions, management of known conditions, and to provide additional information for pregnancies considered for termination [9]. MRI is indicated after inconclusive results with ultrasonography, for a variety of structural abnormalities related to fetal development, particularly for imaging and identification of anomalies of the central nervous system, prior to fetal surgery, and for particularly difficult deliveries [18–21]. Fetal MRI is generally used in addition to ultrasound, primarily due to the relative cost, and can be complicated by fetal motion, wrap-around artifacts limiting the field-of-view, and from multi-slice magnetization transfer from off-resonance artifacts between adjacent slices [22]. Fetal MRI is often performed at a 20-week ultrasound scan [9]. Recently, the MERIDIAN study found that ultrasound provided accurate diagnosis of fetal brain abnormalities at 70% and 64% above and between 18 and 24 weeks, respectively; while fetal MRI in combination with ultrasound increased the accuracy to 92% and 94%, respectively [23]. Clinical radiologists report common referrals to include neurological diagnosis, treatment planning for *in utero* surgery, imaging of congenital masses, and imaging of congenital cardiac defects [24].

2. Fetal MRI sequences and safety for imaging neurodevelopmental and cardiac anomalies

MRI sequence for fetal brain analysis include functional imaging, structural imaging, and diffusion imaging [25]. The predominant sequences used in fetal MRI are single-shot T_2W (SST2W) sequences, such as rapid acquisition with relaxation enhancement (RARE) sequences on Bruker, Single-Shot half-Fourier Turbo Spin Echo (SShTSE) on Philips, Single-shot Fast Spin Echo (SSFSE) on General Electric, and half-Fourier acquisition single-shot turbo spin echo (HASTE) sequences on Siemens, with protocols provided by the MRI vendor [22, 26]. These T_2W sequences are quick enough to be acquired without sedation and are common for neuroanatomical fetal imaging; [9] with other common sequences being T_1W to view hemorrhaging, perfusion MRI, diffusion MRI, and spectroscopy [9, 22]. Default SST2W sequences are generally capable of good image generation with 1x1x4 mm voxel size; using half-Fourier acquisitions, with refocusing pulses with flip angles between 120°-150° [22]. Though difficult to implement, diffusion-weighted imaging (DWI) allows identification of ischemic brain lesions, while T_1W images can provide improvement over T_2W for detection of calcifications, fat, and hemorrhaging [26].

Fetal cardiac sequences are often balanced steady state free precession (bSSFP) and HASTE to encompass small voxel size and reduce acquisition times needed to avoid motion artifacts, with bSSFP being particularly beneficial for imaging blood vessels and cavities containing fluid [26, 27]. Fetal cardiac MRI can be used to view structure, function, vasculature; in addition to performing quantitative MRI measurements including blood flow velocity and oxygen saturation [27]. Blood oxygen level-dependent (BOLD) functional MRI sequences have shown useful for illustrating the improvement of fetal oxygenation during maternal respiratory oxygen therapy for fetuses with impaired cerebral oxygenation resulting from certain types of CHD [28]. Abnormal placenta pathology has been linked with high rates of CHD and is a possible compounding factor for higher severity brain lesions [29]. Neurological implications are not distinct from CHD. Impaired cardiac development is linked with mild brain injury, delayed maturation, shorter gestational age, and smaller brain volumes [30, 31]. Fetal cardiac MRI complications include the smaller size of the fetal heart, lack of gating technologies, and higher heart rate [27].

The primary safety concerns in fetal MRI involve radiofrequency exposure in terms of specific absorption rate (SAR), high acoustic noise, and possibility of peripheral nerve stimulation [22]. MRI is generally considered safe during pregnancy with no evidence of harming the fetus, but is typically not recommended when the fetus is less than about 13 weeks gestational age, and gives best information after completion of organogenesis [22]. The United States Food and Drug Administration (FDA) fetal MRI SAR limit is set at 4 $W.kg^{-1}$ [22, 32]. Fetal MRI scans are usually recommended to be performed at 1.5 T, and as a "golden rule", remain below 25 seconds [20, 22]. 3 T fetal MRI is often used only within research settings because the SAR is four times higher than at 1.5 T; with the upper limit generally at 4 T for research applications [9]. Although, some institutions perform routine 3 T fetal imaging during the late second trimester and throughout the third trimester [33]. Contrast enhancement is not recommended in fetal MRI, thought to enter into the fetal vasculature, passing through the renal system, before emptying into the amniotic fluid [9, 34].

3. Common neurodevelopmental indications for Fetal MRI

Prenatal MRI is most routine for neural abnormalities because of the improved capability for fetal brain scans. In addition to treatment planning of delivery complications, a variety of conditions have high diagnostic rates with fetal MRI, including diagnosis for mild to moderate ventriculomegaly, a variety of neural tube defects, posterior fossa malformations, and twin-to-twin transfusion syndrome [9, 35]. A USA retrospective study for fetal neurology consultations (n = 94) with diagnostic MRI over 14 months reported the most common conditions were posterior fossa malformations, agenesis or dysgenesis of the corpus callosum, congenital acqueductal stenosis, ventriculomegaly, isolated malformations of cortical development, and holoprosencephaly at 19%, 15%, 14%, 11%, 8.5%, and 6%, respectively [36].

Malformations of cortical development are a collection of developmental malformations resulting from disruption during one of the stages of cerebral cortex formation, often causing cognitive impairment, cerebral palsy, and epilepsy. The cortical development occurs in three major stages, including neuronal stem cell proliferation, neuronal migration along radial glial fibers or axons to the developing cerebral cortex, and neuronal organization [37]. Malformations due to abnormal neuronal stem cell proliferation include microcephaly, megalencephaly, and cortical dysplasia. Malformations during neuronal migration and failure for proper cessation of neuronal migration, include: periventricular heterotopia, subcortical band heterotopia, classic lissencephaly, and cobblestone lissencephaly. While, neuronal organization abnormalities include polymicrogyria and schizencephaly [37, 38]. Historically, autopsy or surgical tissue samples were used for diagnosis of these conditions, being difficult to diagnose with ultrasound. MRI has greatly improved the ability to diagnose these conditions during development, rather than in childhood [39]. Retrospective assessment of cortical development malformations has shown high diagnostic accuracy of fetal MRI when compared to postnatal MRI [40].

Ventrigulomegaly is characterized by dilation of the cerebral lateral ventricles during fetal development. Congenital hydrocephalus is a type of ventrigulomegaly that results specifically from increased cerebrospinal fluid pressure, which causes birth defects resulting in abnormally large head size and many other anomalies, and most frequently results from aqueductal stenosis from outlet obstruction in the third ventricle [41, 42]. An illustration of hydrocephalus is shown in **Figure 1**. Characteristic findings seen postnatally are not often observed prenatally, such as aqueduct funneling or obstruction. Fetal MRI diagnostic indicators, for disease severity from aqueductal stenosis, include the extent of enlargement in the lateral and third ventricle, increased size of the third ventricle of inferior recesses, and observance of diverticulum outpouching in the lateral ventricles [43]. A cohort at the national maternity hospital in the Republic of Ireland reported suspected ventriculomegaly as the most common indication for fetal MRI at the facility, with severe ventriculomegaly (exluding termination) showing a 72% survival rate (n = 74) and a 65% rate for cesarean delivery (n = 72) [44].

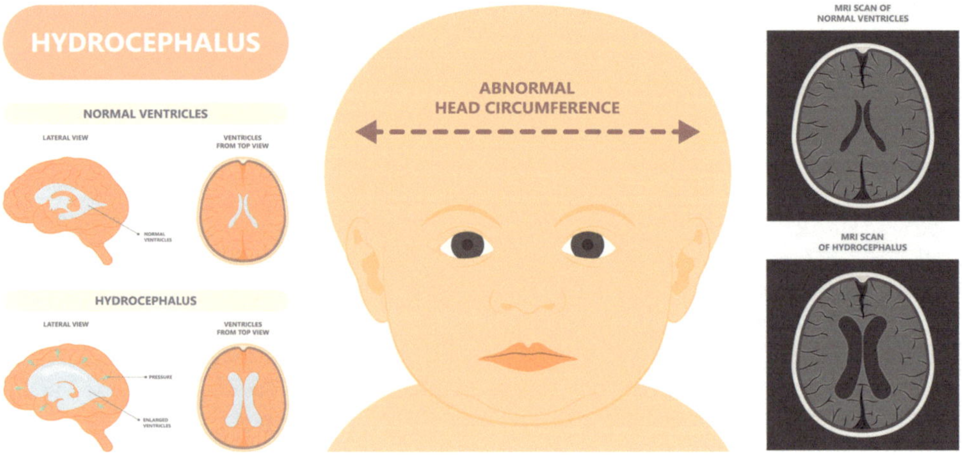

Figure 1.
Illustration of hydrocephalus with MRI. Rumruay/shutterstock.com

Failure of neural tube closure during development results in a variety of neural tube defects, causing spinal anomalies in cases of spinal dysraphism like spina bifida; or cranial anomalies like with anencephaly, characterized by absence of a major portion of the cranium. Though, anencephaly is less indicated for MRI [45]. Distinguishing characteristics of common types of spina bifida are shown in **Figure 2**. Worldwide incidence varies geographically, but estimated on average about 0.1–1% of live births, with anticonvulsants correlating with increased risk, and folic acid associated with reduced risk of neural tube defects [45]. Spinal dysraphism occurs from improper closure of the spinal cord and surrounding membranes during fetal development, and can be classified by open or closed. Closed spina bifida accounts for about 15% of instances, with spina bifida occulta as the most common form, and is usually asymptomatic [33]. Open spina bifida accounts for about 85% of open spinal dysraphisms with myelomenengocele (MMC) and myelocele being predominant, and nearly always presents with Chiari type II malformation [33]. The randomized MOMS trial compared spina bifida outcomes from fetal surgery compared to surgery after delivery, with fetal MRI playing a pivotal role in treatment planning. Outcomes showed fetal surgery for MMC allowed less need for cerebrospinal fluid shunt placement, improved cognitive function in early childhood, though higher risk of preterm birth was observed in the fetal surgery group [33, 46, 47].

Posterior fossa anomalies are characterized by neurodevelopmental malformations in the posterior fossa of the skull cranial cavity. Posterior fossa anomalies are some of the most frequent indications for fetal MRI, occurring in approximately 1 in 5000 live births, encompass a broad spectrum of conditions, and can be categorized as developmental disruptions and malformations [48, 49]. Posterior fossa anomalies include: mega cisterna magna, Blake's pouch cyst, Dandy-Walker malformation, arachnoid cyst, Joubert syndrome, rhombencephalosynapsis, and Chiari malformation [50]. The malformations can present with either an enlarged cyst appearing with abnormally

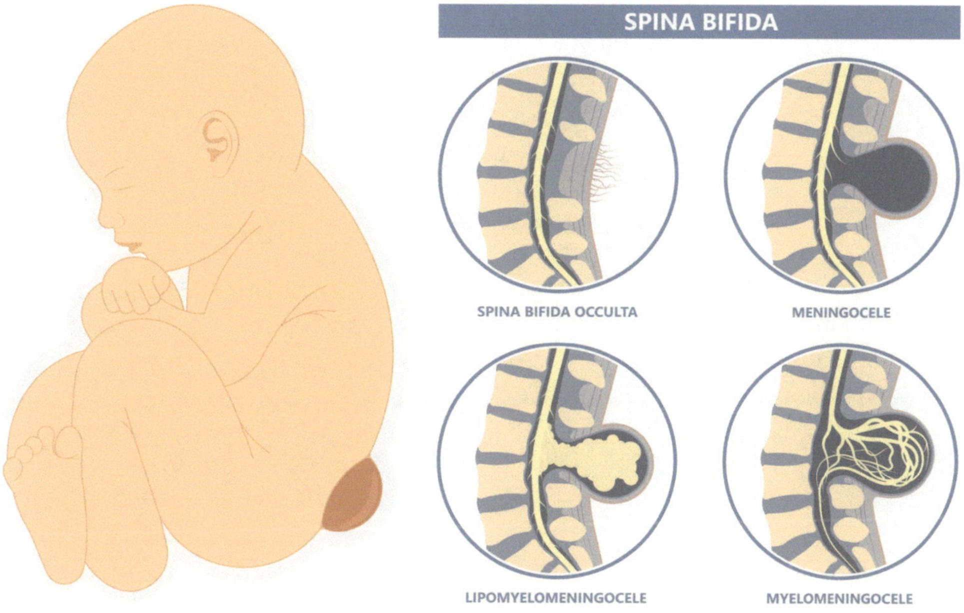

Figure 2.
Comparison of spina bifida subtypes. Rumruay/shutterstock.com

high retrocerebellar fluid, such as in Dandy-Walker malformation, mega cisterna magna, and Blake's pouch cyst. Or the malformations cause an unusually small posterior fossa such as in Dandy-Walker variant [51, 52]. The most common reported malformation is generally Dandy-Walker malformation, presenting with macrocephaly in 90–100% of children within months of delivery [49]. Comparison of fetal MRI and fetal ultrasound images in the diagnosis of Dandy-Walker malformation is shown in **Figure 3**. Prognosis of these conditions is highly influenced by concomitant anomalies, with co-occurring conditions like agenesis and cerebral hypoplasia often resulting in cognitive impairment. Other conditions like mega cisterna magna without hydrocephalus typically result in normal development [50]. In a USA retrospective cohort for ultrasonography referrals for fetal MRI involving posterior fossa anomalies (n = 180), the most common indications for fetal MRI were Dandy-Walker continuum (Dandy-Walker malformation in addition to Dandy-Walker variant) at 42%, mega cisterna magna at 22%, with a change in diagnosis in 70% of cases, and 60% agreement between fetal MRI and postnatal MRI [54].

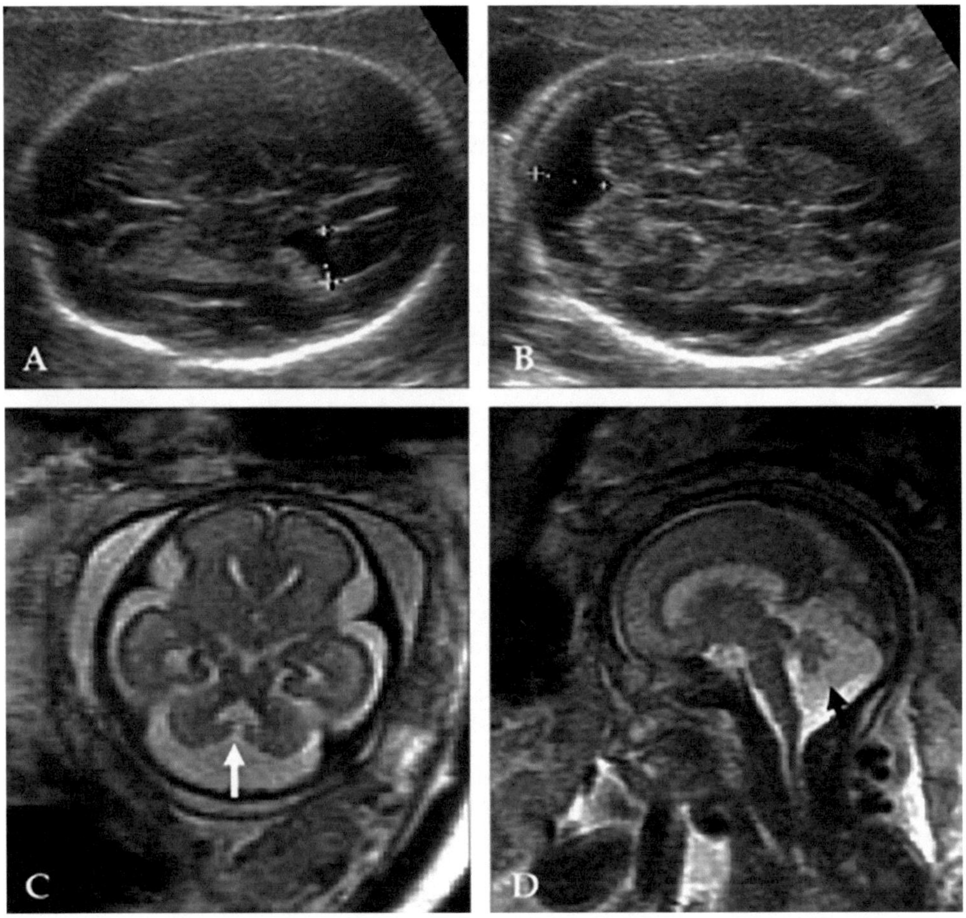

Figure 3.
Dandy-Walker malformation in a 26 week fetus, first suspected as Dandy-Walker variant with ultrasonography, and confirmed as Dandy-Walker malformation with T2W HASTE MRI. A) Ultrasonography illustrating mild ventriculomegaly B) ultrasonography image illustrating cisterna magna that is abnormally large. C) MRI image illustrating direct connection between the cisterna magna and 4th ventricle. D) Sagittal MRI of abnormally large posterior fossa. Reprint Sohn et al., 2008 under CC BY-NC 3.0 [53].

The corpus callosum is a white matter commissural nerve tract, connecting cortical regions of left and right hemispheres, and composed of myelinated axons that allow action potential propagation [55]. The corpus callosum forms between gestational weeks 11–22, is composed of five distinct regions, and hyperplasia or hypoplasia of these regions is termed callosal dysgenesis, while total absence is deemed callosal agenesis [56]. Agenesis of the corpus callosum rarely occurs in complete isolation, and generally occurs in combination with other disorders. MRI can provide more detail for the extent of the condition than ultrasonography alone [55]. This allows confirmation that the corpus callosum is intact and visualization of co-occurring and associated malformations [9]. Diffusion tensor imaging and fiber tractography in developing research applications has greatly improved the understanding of the neuronal tracts of the corpus callosum, and complications associated with different degrees of agenesis [55]. Tractography has allowed characterization of normal developmental patterns for the nerve bundles of the corpus callosum with increasing gestational age, showing an increase in volume and fractional anisotropy, with a decrease in apparent diffusion coefficient [57].

In twin-to-twin transfusion syndrome, unequal blood supply to the fetuses leads to demise of one twin. Untreated cases have dismal survival rates [58]. The condition indicates diagnostic fetal MRI due to improved capabilities over ultrasonography for identifying ischemic lesions and neurodevelopmental abnormalities. The condition often warrants intervention including serial amniocentesis or *in utero* fetoscopic laser ablation of the blood supply of the surviving twin [18]. This condition is hypothesized to be the cause of death for two fetuses found in the tomb of King Tutankhamen, whom are believed to be his two stillborn twin daughters [59, 60].

4. Common cardiac indications for Fetal MRI

Ultrasonography is the primary imaging modality for monitoring and diagnosis in both congenital and acquired pediatric heart disease and antenatal complications [61]. Ultrasonography and MRI have been determined safe for fetal imaging, but suggested to be used prudently, with common concerns and power limits due to potential tissue heating and acoustic damage [62]. Fetal cardiac MRI can improve outcomes by allowing earlier preparation of treatment procedures [63]. The American Heart Association (AHA) and British Association of Perinatal Medicine (BAPM) suggest neonatal MRI for newborn patients with high-risk CHD in combination of evidence for intracranial hemorrhaging or parenchymal brain trauma, though not recommended for routine use for CHD [9].

CHD is the most common form of congenital abnormalities, occurring in about 0.6–0.8% of live births, with as much as half of the patients requiring open-heart surgery, and is associated with high rates of neurodevelopmental problems [9]. CHD is associated with high neonatal morbidity, particularly in preterm infants [64]. Some of the most common congenital heart abnormalities include atrial septal defects, ventricular septal defects, Tetralogy of Fallot, patent ductus arteriosus, and pulmonary stenosis [65, 66]. A depiction of several types of congenital heart defects is shown in **Figure 4**. Ventricular septal defects are the most common congenital cardiac anomaly, often requiring surgical repair, though a high percentage will also spontaneously close with age [66–68].

Prenatal cardiac MRI for CHD has generally been limited to a research setting [69]. This has been due to factors including inability to perform electrocardiogram gating,

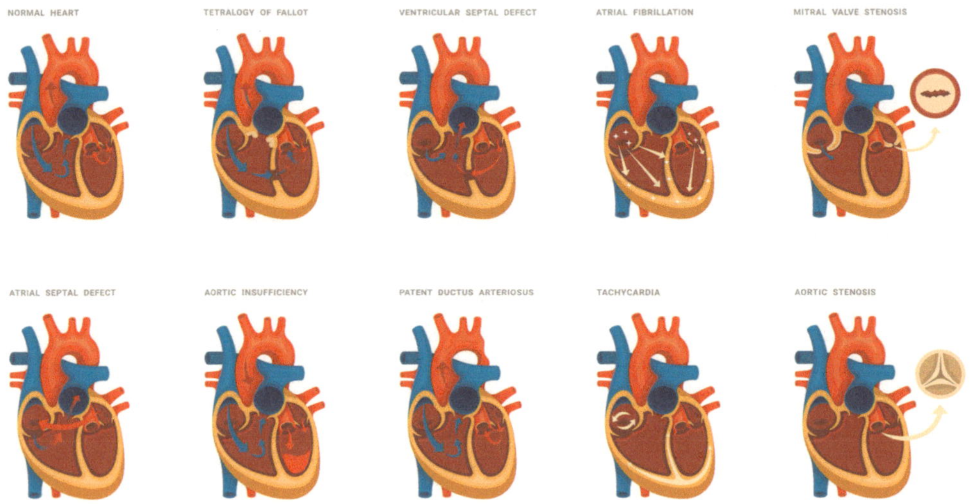

Figure 4.
Illustration of common congenital heart defects. N.Style/shutterstock.com

fetal motion, insufficient safety data, and the relatively small size of the features of the fetal heart [70, 71]. Prenatal cardiac MRI allows evaluation of cardiac anatomy, cardiac function, vascular anatomy, flow quantification, and oxygen content [69].

Recent advances has allowed image reconstruction techniques to obtain high-resolution 3D MRI of the fetal heart to assess for congenital heart defects. 3D MRI with motion-corrected image registration was shown in a cohort study to significantly increase visualization and diagnosis of major fetal vascular heart defects in late-gestational age fetuses, when compared to 2D MRI [72]. Additionally, Doppler ultrasonography has shown capable of performing cardiac gating of the fetal heart to generate high-quality bSSFP cine images [73].

A cohort study reported the use of a non-contrast velocity-selective arterial spin labelling (VSASL) sequence to assess placental perfusion in fetuses with CHD compared to fetuses without CHD [74]. The study found decreased global perfusion and increased variation of regional perfusion were linked to increasing gestational age in CHD fetuses. The results also suggest that early placental perfusion may increase to compensate for the heart defect.

A Chinese retrospective study reported findings in 1379 confirmed cases for fetal cardiac MRI from 2005 to 2019, referred after echocardiography could not show the four cardiac chambers in addition to ventricular outflow [75]. Imaging sequences were SSFP, real-time cine SSFP, non-gated phase contrast sequences, and SSTSE. The findings were normal in 92.5% of cases, 5.1% presented with CHD, and 2.4% were diagnosed with an alternative heart condition. In the CHD cases, 56% received correct diagnosis with MRI, which was similar to other studies, as prenatal detection rates for CHD for patients that eventually underwent congenital heart surgery, have tended to be low and less than 50% [76].

5. MRI in Fetal surgery

Most conditions are best treated when the fetus is delivered at term; however, certain instances warrant the use of *in utero* fetal surgery [77]. Traditionally, this has been limited to cases of high likelihood of mortality for the fetus without intervention, as the technique is high-risk of morbidity and mortality to the mother. More recently, fetal surgery has allowed interventions for improved life quality [78]. MRI has proved beneficial for fetal surgery planning when indicated for conditions, including fetal tracheolaryngeal airway obstruction, congenital diaphragmatic hernia, congenital pulmonary airway malformation, myelomeningocele spina bifida, congenital heart defects, and lower urinary tract obstruction [77, 78]. Additionally, fetal MRI has shown useful to assess effects of fetal myelomeningocele repair, by comparison of before and after MRI images to uncomplicated fetuses of the same gestational age [79]. Also, MRI has shown beneficial in patient selection for fetal intervention prior to EXIT delivery in congenital high airway obstructive syndrome [80].

6. Fetal MRI for pregnancy complications

Again, ultrasonography is recommended as the first imaging modality, but MRI is often indicated in a variety of maternal obstetric and non-obstetric complications during pregnancy, including placental adhesive disorders, placental abruption, prognosis of uterine rupture, restricted circulation in placental bed disorders, placental insufficiency, acute appendicitis during pregnancy, prediction of preterm labor, ovarian cysts, and urolithiasis [18, 81]. Additionally, MRI is indicated in treatment planning for difficult deliveries, such as those that require the EXIT procedure due to fetal airway obstruction [9]. Moreover, the technique has proved useful in risk scoring for massive intraoperative hemorrhage in patients with previous cesarean sections and exhibiting placenta previa and accreta [82]. Fetal MRI was recently used in a randomized control trial to assess fetal neurodevelopmental improvement for supplemental pomegranate juice in pregnancies with intrauterine growth restriction [83].

7. Fetal MRI for viral infections

Prenatal MRI is useful for diagnosis of complications associated with maternal viral infections, including the more recent complications associated with SARS-CoV-2 infection.

7.1 Prenatal MRI for complications from viral infections other than SARS-CoV-2

A variety of fetal complications arising from viral infection can be imaged with MRI, particularly for identifying neurological sequelae, but also for conditions including fetal ascites, hydrops, cardiomegaly, and pericardial effusion [84]. Fetal MRI can be indicated for diagnosis of suspected neurotropic pathogens, such as cytomegalovirus, Zika virus, and toxoplasmosis [85–88]. Cytomegalovirus is a member of the Herpesviridae family, the most common vertically transmitted congenital viral infection, and the most common infection that results in deafness and intellectual disability in children [89, 90]. MRI and ultrasonography can identify fetal brain lesions resulting from cytomegalovirus infection. MRI diagnosis of infection-related complications allows the possibility of treatment planning for investigational therapies, including antiviral therapy such as Valaciclovir or hyperimmunoglobulin therapy, in the neonates and in fetuses [18, 91, 92].

7.2 Prenatal MRI for complications involving the SARS-CoV-2 virus

SARS-CoV-2 is a positive sense, lipid-enveloped, single-stranded, RNA coronavirus that causes both upper and lower respiratory tract infection, which can result in severe pulmonary inflammation and pneumonia, in a condition denoted human coronavirus disease or more recently COVID-19 [93–95].

SARS-CoV-2 relies upon two types of entry pathways to enter cells through the interaction of the virion spike (S) protein with angiotensin-converting enzyme 2 (ACE2), with release of internal RNA within the cell occurring after cleavage of the S-protein subunits [95]. After binding to ACE2, if transmembrane protease serine 2 (TMPRSS2) is present on the cell surface, the cleavage event occurs through TMPRSS2 and furin, initiating membrane fusion and fusion pore formation on the cell membrane, and release of viral RNA into the cellular cytoplasm [95]. Alternatively, if little or no TMPRSS2 is present on the surface, the clathrin-mediated endocytosis occurs and the virus is internalized intracellularly within endolysosomes, followed by a cathepsin-cleavage event within the endosome, resulting in membrane fusion and release of the viral RNA into the cell cytoplasm [95].

The BNT162b2 (Pfizer, BioNTech) and Spikevax (Moderna, NIAID) are both mRNA-based vaccines that encompass an mRNA strand encoding the spike protein for the original Wuhan-Hu-1 strain, in a liposomal mRNA-lipid nanoparticle, which has a notable ability for large-scale production [95, 96]. The vaccine causes cells to encode the vaccine mRNA to produce spike proteins that are then expressed into the cell membrane. This causes an antibody response that identify these spike protein antigens as a foreign body, stimulating a B-cell and T-cell lymphocyte response to produce antibodies that will tag future spike proteins from SARS-CoV-2 viremia [97]. The viral mutations of these spike protein antigens result in reduced efficacy of the vaccines to induce a immunogenic response. Because mRNA vaccines require antibody neutralization of viremia, mutations in the spike proteins can allow variants to exhibit resistance to the vaccines, potentially causing more severe infections, higher transmissibility, and the possibility of re-infection in vaccinated individuals [98, 99].

A prospective U.K. cohort found 0.5% incidence of SARS-CoV-2 infection during pregnancy that required hospital admission (n = 427) [100]. Of the patients that delivered or experienced pregnancy loss at the time of the article (n = 262), 10% required intensive care unit (ICU) admission and death occurred in 1.2%. From the SARS-CoV-2 positive pregnancies with live born births, 59% had cesarean deliveries and 25% of neonates were admitted to the neonatal intensive care unit (NICU). Preterm delivery occurred in 25% of cases, most of which were induced labor due to COVID-19 complications, and 5% of neonates were COVID-19 positive within 12 hours of birth.

Pregnant women are at high risk of developing severe COVID-19 compared to non-pregnant women, in terms of adjusted risk. Comparing COVID-19 positive pregnancies with non-COVID-19 pregnancies, studies have observed a factor of 3 increase in ICU admissions and invasive intubation with mechanical ventilation, a factor of 2.4 increase in odds for extracorporeal membrane oxygenation, and 70% increase in death [101]. Severe COVID-19 complications are linked with increased rates of preterm birth, hypertensive disorders, and cesarean births [101]. Studies have linked COVID-19 with significant increased mortality for mothers post-delivery and in neonates; particularly for symptomatic patients and those with underlying comorbidities [102, 103]. Neonatal outcomes have been reported as generally favorable, with about half of cases being asymptomatic; though, neonates and children less than one year of age are thought to possibly exhibit higher risk of acute respiratory failure than other children [104].

Risk of vertical transmission of SARS-CoV-2 from mother to fetus is considered low, with the primary transmission to the neonate being through horizontal transmission [101, 105]. Although, at least one case study has confirmed vertical transplacental transmission [106]. There is little evidence for transmission of SARS-CoV-2 through breast milk to the neonate, but pasteurization has been shown to inactivate the SARS-CoV-2 virus and might be considered in specific cases for positive SARS-CoV-2 mothers [101, 105, 107]. Transmission between members of the same family cluster is the primary means of infection from SARS-CoV-2 in children [108]. Infection in children and adolescents has tended to result in milder symptoms and good prognosis, in general [109].

The American College of Radiology (ACR) has suggested limiting the use of MRI to only cases that are absolutely necessary, for COVID-19 positive patients and those suspected of infection [110]. The use of fetal MRI for COVID-19 positive mothers does not have a common indication for routine use and has mostly been reported as case studies or small cohorts. Fetal MRI has been used in cohorts to assess possible neurodevelopmental damage in the fetuses of mothers with SARS-CoV-2 infection during early pregnancy, with results showing no abnormal findings [111]. However, a case study of *in utero* transplacental transmission did reveal white matter damage in a neonate, causing placental inflammation in the mother, and ill-effects in the neonate, including bilateral gliosis and white cortical matter damage on MRI from which the infant slowly recovered [106]. A cohort of 34 pregnant patients assessed lung volume with fetal MRI for complications associated with infection in mildly symptomatic SARS-CoV-2 positive mothers. The study found that the fetal lung volume to body weight ratio was noticeably reduced, particularly when the infection occurred during the third trimester; though neonates did not exhibit respiratory distress [112]. Many cases studies are reported for MRI diagnosis of non-obstetric complications of pregnant COVID-19 patients for a variety of common complications, such as stroke [113] and appendicitis [114].

A significant increase in obstetrical complications in COVID-19 has been observed, compared to non-COVID-19 pregnancies. Studies have shown higher rates of fetal deaths, maternal deaths, ICU admissions, preterm births, and cesarean deliveries. These outcomes highlight the benefit of vaccination during pregnancy, to reduce the risk of maternal and fetal complications [101].

8. Conclusions

Prenatal MRI offers useful complementary diagnostic information to ultrasonography, particularly for neurodevelopmental complications. The technique can be used for diagnosis, for guiding treatment decisions, and to counsel parents for scenarios like potential termination. MRI has been determined safe for fetal health, though low field strengths and non-contrast imaging are generally used, as these scenarios are lower risk to the fetus. MRI can improve diagnostic accuracy for neurodevelopmental and cardiac anomalies when used in conjunction with ultrasonography, but factors like additional cost limits the number of indications for prenatal diagnosis. Studies have shown increased rates of pregnancy-related complications in patients infected with SARS-CoV-2 during pregnancy. Although, studies with fetal MRI for assessing fetal developmental complications due to maternal COVID-19 has been limited, but results have been reported in case studies and small cohorts.

Acknowledgements

Thanks to the Center for Biomedical Imaging and the Image-guided Interventions Laboratory for supporting the development of this manuscript. Thanks to Dr. Daniela Dumitriu LaGrange for reviewing the manuscript and suggesting improvements.

Author details

Ryan Holman
Image Guided Interventions Laboratory, Department of Radiology, University of Geneva, Switzerland

*Address all correspondence to: ryan.holman@unige.ch

References

[1] Lawn JE, Blencowe H, Oza S, You D, Lee AC, Waiswa P, et al. Every Newborn: Progress, priorities, and potential beyond survival. Lancet. 2014; **384**(9938):189-205

[2] Oza S, Lawn JE, Hogan DR, Mathers C, Cousens SN. Neonatal cause-of-death estimates for the early and late neonatal periods for 194 countries: 2000-2013. Bulletin of the World Health Organization. 2014;**93**:19-28

[3] Purisch SE, Gyamfi-Bannerman C. Epidemiology of preterm birth. In: Seminars in Perinatology. Vol. 41. Amsterdam: Elsevier; 2021. pp. 387-391

[4] Blencowe H, Cousens S, Chou D, Oestergaard M, Say L, Moller AB, et al. Born too soon: The global epidemiology of 15 million preterm births. Reproductive Health. 2013;**10**(1):1-14

[5] Simen-Kapeu A, Seale AC, Wall S, Nyange C, Qazi SA, Moxon SG, et al. Treatment of neonatal infections: A multi-country analysis of health system bottlenecks and potential solutions. BMC Pregnancy and Childbirth. 2015;**15**(2):S6

[6] Heron MP. Deaths: Leading causes for 2017. National Vital Statistics Reports. 2019;**68**:1-77

[7] Moshiro R, Mdoe P, Perlman JM. A global view of neonatal asphyxia and resuscitation. Frontiers in Pediatrics. 2019;**7**:1-6

[8] van der Linde D, Konings EEM, Slager MA, Witsenburg M, Helbing WA, Takkenberg JJM, et al. Birth prevalence of congenital heart disease worldwide. Journal of the American College of Cardiology. 2011;**58**(21): 2241-2247

[9] British Association of Perinatal Medicine. Fetal and neonatal brain magnetic resonance imaging: Clinical indications, acquisitions and reporting—A framework for practice. A Framework for Practice. 2016

[10] Kazemi M, Salehi M, Kheirollahi M. Down syndrome: Current status, challenges and future perspectives. International Journal of Molecular and Cellular Medicine. 2016;**5**(3):125-133

[11] Sahmat A, Gunasekaran R, Mohd-Zin SW, Balachandran L, Thong MK, Engkasan JP, et al. The prevalence and distribution of spina bifida in a single major referral Center in Malaysia. Frontiers in Pediatrics. 2017;**5**

[12] Greene NDE, Copp AJ. Neural tube defects. Annual Review of Neuroscience. 2014;**37**(1):221-242

[13] Paslaru FG, Panaitescu AM, Iancu G, Veduta A, Gica N, Paslaru AC, et al. Myelomeningocele surgery over the 10 years following the MOMS trial: A systematic review of outcomes in prenatal versus postnatal surgical repair. Medicina. 2021;**57**(7):1-13

[14] Dubois J, Dehaene-Lambertz G, Kulikova S, Poupon C, Hüppi PS, Hertz-Pannier L. The early development of brain white matter: A review of imaging studies in fetuses, newborns and infants. Neuroscience. 2014;**276**:48-71

[15] Yan W. Womb zoom: What advances in fetal and newborn imaging have revealed. Nature Medicine. 2017; **23**(3):270-272

[16] Andescavage NN, du Plessis A, McCarter R, Serag A, Evangelou I, Vezina G, et al. Complex trajectories of

brain development in the healthy human Fetus. Cerebral Cortex. 2016;**27**(11): 5274-5283

[17] Vasung L, Lepage C, Rados M, Pletikos M, Goldman JS, Richiardi J, et al. Quantitative and qualitative analysis of transient Fetal compartments during prenatal human brain development. Frontiers in Neuroanatomy. 2016;**10**:1-17

[18] Brunelli R, Masselli G. Clinical Indications to MRI in Pregnancy, MRI of Fetal and Maternal Diseases in Pregnancy. Cham: Springer; 2016. pp. 1-20

[19] Saleem SN. Fetal MRI: An approach to practice: A review. Journal of Advanced Research. 2014;**5**(5):507-523

[20] Prayer D, Malinger G, Brugger PC, Cassady C, De Catte L, De Keersmaecker B, et al. ISUOG practice guidelines: Performance of fetal magnetic resonance imaging. Ultrasound in Obstetrics & Gynecology. 2017;**49**(5): 671-680

[21] Levine D. Fetal magnetic resonance imaging. The Journal of Maternal-Fetal & Neonatal Medicine. 2004;**15**(2):85-94

[22] Gholipour A, Estroff JA, Barnewolt CE, Robertson RL, Grant PE, Gagoski B, et al. Fetal MRI: A technical update with educational aspirations. Concepts in Magnetic Resonance Part A. 2014;**43**(6):237-266

[23] Griffiths PD, Bradburn M, Campbell MJ, Cooper CL, Graham R, Jarvis D, et al. Use of MRI in the diagnosis of fetal brain abnormalities in utero (MERIDIAN): A multicentre, prospective cohort study. Lancet. 2017; **389**(10068):538-546

[24] Saleem SN. How to read and to report a Fetal MRI examination. In: MRI of Fetal and Maternal Diseases in Pregnancy. Cham: Springer; 2016. pp. 57-74

[25] Rousseau F, Studholme C, Jardri R, Thomason ME. In vivo human fetal brain analysis using MR imaging. In: Fetal Development. Cham: Springer; 2016. pp. 407-427

[26] Koberlein G, Hosseinzadeh K, Anthony EY. Fetal MR imaging: Protocols and anatomy. In: MRI of Fetal and Maternal Diseases in Pregnancy. Cham: Springer; 2016. pp. 35-56

[27] Roy CW, van Amerom JFP, Marini D, Seed M, Macgowan CK. Fetal cardiac MRI: A review of technical advancements. Topics in Magnetic Resonance Imaging. 2019;**28**(5):235-244

[28] You W, Andescavage NN, Kapse K, Donofrio MT, Jacobs M, Limperopoulos C. Hemodynamic responses of the placenta and brain to maternal Hyperoxia in Fetuses with congenital heart disease by using blood oxygen—Level dependent MRI. Radiology. 2020;**294**(1):141-148

[29] Schlatterer SD, Murnick J, Jacobs M, White L, Donofrio MT, Limperopoulos C. Placental pathology and neuroimaging correlates in neonates with congenital heart disease. Scientific Reports. 2019; **9**(1):1-11

[30] Brossard-Racine M, Du Plessis AJ, Vezina G, Robertson R, Bulas D, Evangelou IE, et al. Prevalence and Spectrum of In utero structural brain abnormalities in Fetuses with complex congenital heart disease. American Journal of Neuroradiology. 2014;**35**(8): 1593-1599

[31] Limperopoulos C, Tworetzky W, McElhinney DB, Newburger JW, Brown DW, Robertson RL, et al. Brain

volume and metabolism in Fetuses with congenital heart disease. Circulation. 2010;**121**(1):26-33

[32] Pugash D, Brugger PC, Bettelheim D, Prayer D. Prenatal ultrasound and fetal MRI: The comparative value of each modality in prenatal diagnostics. European Journal of Radiology. 2008;**68**(2):214-226

[33] Shekdar KV. MRI of fetal spine and extremities. In: MRI of Fetal and Maternal Diseases in Pregnancy. Cham: Springer; 2016. pp. 139-158

[34] Seely JM. MRI-guided biopsy procedures. In: Interventional Breast Procedures: A Practical Approach. Cham: Springer; 2019. pp. 85-146

[35] Reddy UM, Abuhamad AZ, Levine D, Saade GR. Fetal imaging: Executive summary of a joint Eunice Kennedy Shriver National Institute of Child Health and Human Development, Society for Maternal-Fetal Medicine, American Institute of Ultrasound in Medicine, American College of Obstetricians and Gynecologists, American College of Radiology, Society for Pediatric Radiology, and Society of Radiologists in ultrasound Fetal imaging workshop. American Journal of Obstetrics and Gynecology. 2014;**210**(5): 387-397

[36] Arroyo MS, Hopkin RJ, Nagaraj UD, Kline-Fath B, Venkatesan C. Fetal brain MRI findings and neonatal outcome of common diagnosis at a tertiary care center. Journal of Perinatology. 2019; **39**(8):1072-1077

[37] Barkovich AJ, Kuzniecky RI, Jackson GD, Guerrini R, Dobyns WB. A developmental and genetic classification for malformations of cortical development. Neurology. 2005;**65**(12): 1873-1887

[38] Pang T, Atefy R, Sheen V. Malformations of cortical development. The Neurologist. 2008;**14**(3):181-191

[39] Severino M, Geraldo AF, Utz N, Tortora D, Pogledic I, Klonowski W, et al. Definitions and classification of malformations of cortical development: Practical guidelines. Brain. 2020; **143**(10):2874-2894

[40] Glenn OA, Cuneo AA, Barkovich AJ, Hashemi Z, Bartha AI, Xu D. Malformations of cortical development: Diagnostic accuracy of Fetal MR imaging. Radiology. 2012;**263**(3):843-855

[41] Kahle KT, Kulkarni AV, Limbrick DD, Warf BC. Hydrocephalus in children. The Lancet. 2016; **387**(10020):788-799

[42] Scola E, Triulzi F. Ventriculomegaly. In: Perinatal Neuroradiology: From the Fetus to the Newborn. Milan: Springer; 2016. pp. 201-220

[43] Heaphy-Henault KJ, Guimaraes CV, Mehollin-Ray AR, Cassady CI, Zhang W, Desai NK, et al. Congenital Aqueductal stenosis: Findings at Fetal MRI that accurately predict a postnatal diagnosis. American Journal of Neuroradiology. 2018;**39**(5):942-948

[44] Start AO, Ryan GA, Cathcart B, Hughes H, Higgins S, Corcoran S, et al. Severe fetal ventriculomegaly: Fetal morbidity and mortality, caesarean delivery rates and obstetrical challenges in a large prospective cohort. Prenatal Diagnosis. 2022;**42**(1):109-117

[45] Zugazaga Cortazar A, MartÃ-n Martinez C, Duran Feliubadalo C, Bella Cueto MR, Serra L. Magnetic resonance imaging in the prenatal diagnosis of neural tube defects. Insights Into Imaging. 2013;**4**(2):225-237

[46] Adzick NS, Thom EA, Spong CY, Brock JW, Burrows PK, Johnson MP, et al. A randomized trial of prenatal versus postnatal repair of myelomeningocele. The New England Journal of Medicine. 2011;**364**(11): 993-1004

[47] Tulipan N, Wellons JC, Thom EA, Gupta N, Sutton LN, Burrows PK, et al. Prenatal surgery for myelomeningocele and the need for cerebrospinal fluid shunt placement. Journal of Neurosurgery. Pediatrics. 2015;**16**(6): 613-620

[48] Mahalingam HV, Rangasami R, Seshadri S, Suresh I. Imaging spectrum of posterior fossa anomalies on foetal magnetic resonance imaging with an algorithmic approach to diagnosis. Polish Journal of Radiology. 2021;**86**:e183-e194

[49] Bosemani T, Orman G, Boltshauser E, Tekes A, Huisman TAGM, Poretti A. Congenital abnormalities of the Posterior Fossa. Radiographics. 2015;**35**(1):200-220

[50] Chapman T, Mahalingam S, Ishak GE, Nixon JN, Siebert J, Dighe MK. Diagnostic imaging of posterior fossa anomalies in the fetus and neonate: Part 2, posterior fossa disorders. Clinical Imaging. 2015;**39**(2):167-175

[51] Shekdar K. Posterior fossa malformations. Semin Ultrasound CT MRI. 2011;**32**(3):228-241

[52] Chapman T, Mahalingam S, Ishak GE, Nixon JN, Siebert J, Dighe MK. Diagnostic imaging of posterior fossa anomalies in the fetus and neonate: Part 1, normal anatomy and classification of anomalies. Clinical Imaging. 2015;**39**(1):1-8

[53] Sohn YS, Kim MJ, Kwon JY, Kim YH, Park YW. The usefulness of fetal MRI for prenatal diagnosis. Yonsei Medical Journal. 2007;**48**(4):671-677

[54] Schlatterer SD, Sanapo L, du Plessis AJ, Whitehead MT, Mulkey SB. The role of Fetal MRI for suspected anomalies of the Posterior Fossa. Pediatric Neurology. 2021;**117**:10-18

[55] Edwards TJ, Sherr EH, Barkovich AJ, Richards LJ. Clinical, genetic and imaging findings identify new causes for corpus callosum development syndromes. Brain. 2014;**137**(6):1579-1613

[56] Alford RE, Bailey AA, Twickler DM. Fetal central nervous system. In: MRI of Fetal and Maternal Diseases in Pregnancy. Cham: Springer; 2016. pp. 91-118

[57] Jaimes C, Machado-Rivas F, Afacan O, Khan S, Marami B, Ortinau CM, et al. In vivo characterization of emerging white matter microstructure in the fetal brain in the third trimester. Human Brain Mapping. 2020;**41**(12):3177-3185

[58] Mason J, Sidebottom N. Twin to twin transfusion syndrome. Newborn and Infant Nursing Reviews. 2007;**7**(4): 193-196. Fetal Therapeutics

[59] Hawass Z, Saleem SN. Mummified daughters of king Tutankhamun: Archeologic and CT studies. American Journal of Roentgenology. 2011;**197**(5): W829-W836

[60] Chamberlain G. Two babies that could have changed world history. The Historian. 2001;**72**:6-10

[61] Lai WW, Geva T, Shirali GS, Frommelt PC, Humes RA, Brook MM, et al. Guidelines and standards for performance of a pediatric echocardiogram: A report from the task force of the Pediatric Council of the

American Society of echocardiography. Journal of the American Society of Echocardiography. 2006;**19**(12): 1413-1430

[62] American College of Obstetricians and Gynecologists. Guidelines for diagnostic imaging during pregnancy and lactation. Committee opinion No. 723. Obstetrics and Gynecology. 2017; **130**(4):e210ee216

[63] Loomba RS, Chandrasekar S, Shah PH, Sanan P. The developing role of fetal magnetic resonance imaging in the diagnosis of congenital cardiac anomalies: A systematic review. Annals of Pediatric Cardiology. 2011;**4**(2): 172-176

[64] Steurer MA, Baer RJ, Chambers CD, Costello J, Franck LS, McKenzie-Sampson S, et al. Mortality and major neonatal morbidity in preterm infants with serious congenital heart disease. The Journal of Pediatrics. 2021;**239**: 110-116.e3

[65] Mohammad N, Shaikh S, Memon S, Das H. Spectrum of heart disease in children under 5 years of age at Liaquat university hospital, Hyderabad, Pakistan. Indian Heart Journal. 2014; **66**(1):145-149

[66] Cavalcante JL, Lalude OO, Schoenhagen P, Lerakis S. Cardiovascular magnetic resonance imaging for structural and Valvular heart disease interventions. JACC. Cardiovascular Interventions. 2016;**9**(5): 399-425

[67] Turner S, Hunter S, Wyllie J. The natural history of ventricular septal defects. Archives of Disease in Childhood. 1999;**81**(5):413-416

[68] Roguin N, Du ZD, Barak M, Nasser N, Hershkowitz S, Milgram E. High prevalence of muscular ventricular septal defect in neonates. Journal of the American College of Cardiology. 1995; **26**(6):1545-1548

[69] Pushparajah K, Lloyd DF. Role of Fetal cardiac magnetic resonance imaging. In: Fetal Cardiology. Cham: Springer; 2018. pp. 189-197

[70] Donofrio MT, Moon-Grady AJ, Hornberger LK, Copel JA, Sklansky MS, Abuhamad A, et al. Diagnosis and treatment of Fetal cardiac disease. Circulation. 2014;**129**(21):2183-2242

[71] Prakash A, Powell AJ, Geva T. Multimodality noninvasive imaging for assessment of congenital heart disease. Circulation. Cardiovascular Imaging. 2010;**3**(1):112-125

[72] Lloyd DFA, Pushparajah K, Simpson JM, van Amerom JFP, van Poppel MPM, Schulz A, et al. Three-dimensional visualisation of the fetal heart using prenatal MRI with motion-corrected slice-volume registration: A prospective, single-Centre cohort study. Lancet. 2019;**393**(10181):1619-1627

[73] Kording F, Yamamura J, de Sousa MT, Ruprecht C, Hedström E, Aletras AH, et al. Dynamic fetal cardiovascular magnetic resonance imaging using Doppler ultrasound gating [journal article]. Journal of Cardiovascular Magnetic Resonance. 2018;**20**(1):17

[74] Zun Z, Zaharchuk G, Andescavage NN, Donofrio MT, Limperopoulos C. Non-invasive placental perfusion imaging in pregnancies complicated by Fetal heart disease using velocity-selective arterial spin Labeled MRI. Scientific Reports. 2017;7(1):16126

[75] Dong SZ, Zhu M, Ji H, Ren JY, Liu K. Fetal cardiac MRI: A single center

experience over 14-years on the potential utility as an adjunct to fetal technically inadequate echocardiography. Scientific Reports. 2020;**10**(1):12373

[76] Quartermain MD, Pasquali SK, Hill KD, Goldberg DJ, Huhta JC, Jacobs JP, et al. Variation in prenatal diagnosis of congenital heart disease in infants. Pediatrics. 2015;**136**(2):e378-e385

[77] Helal AA. Principles of Fetal surgery. In: Shehata S, editor. Pediatric Surgery, Flowcharts and Clinical Algorithms. Rijeka: IntechOpen; 2019. pp. 1-20

[78] Cozzi DA, Ceccanti S. 5. In: Masselli G, editor. Fetal MRI: Contribution to Perinatal Management and Fetal Surgical Treatment of Congenital Anomalies. Cham: Springer International Publishing; 2016. pp. 75-87

[79] Mufti N, Aertsen M, Ebner M, Fidon L, Patel P, Rahman MBA, et al. Cortical spectral matching and shape and volume analysis of the fetal brain pre- and post-fetal surgery for spina bifida: A retrospective study. Neuroradiology. 2021;**63**(10):1721-1734

[80] Saadai P, Jelin EB, Nijagal A, Schecter SC, Hirose S, MacKenzie TC, et al. Long-term outcomes after fetal therapy for congenital high airway obstructive syndrome. Journal of Pediatric Surgery. 2012;**47**(6):1095-1100

[81] Gatta G, Di Grezia G, Cuccurullo V, Sardu C, Iovino F, Comune R, et al. MRI in pregnancy and precision medicine: A review from literature. Journal of Personalized Medicine. 2022;**12**(1):1-16

[82] Chen D, Xu J, Ye P, Li M, Duan X, Zhao F, et al. Risk scoring system with MRI for intraoperative massive hemorrhage in placenta previa and accreta. Journal of Magnetic Resonance Imaging. 2020;**51**(3):947-958

[83] Ross MM, Cherkerzian S, Mikulis ND, Turner D, Robinson J, Inder TE, et al. A randomized controlled trial investigating the impact of maternal dietary supplementation with pomegranate juice on brain injury in infants with IUGR. Scientific Reports. 2021;**11**(1):3569

[84] Triulzi F, Doneda C, Parazzini C, Righini A. Congenital infections. In: Perinatal Neuroradiology: From the Fetus to the Newborn. Milano: Springer Milan; 2016. pp. 221-235

[85] Barkovich AJ, Girard N. Fetal brain infections. Child's Nervous System. 2003;**19**(7–8):501-507

[86] Doneda C, Parazzini C, Righini A, Rustico M, Tassis B, Fabbri E, et al. Early cerebral lesions in cytomegalovirus infection: Prenatal MR imaging. Radiology. 2010;**255**(2):613-621

[87] Guillemette-Artur P, Besnard M, Eyrolle-Guignot D, Jouannic JM, Garel C. Prenatal brain MRI of fetuses with Zika virus infection. Pediatric Radiology. 2016;**46**(7):1032-1039

[88] Driggers RW, Ho CY, Korhonen EM, Kuivanen S, Jääskeläinen AJ, Smura T, et al. Zika virus infection with prolonged maternal viremia and Fetal brain abnormalities. The New England Journal of Medicine. 2016;**374**(22): 2142-2151

[89] Britt WJ, Goodrum F. Congenital human cytomegalovirus infection and the enigma of maternal immunity. Journal of Virology. 2017;**91**(15):e02392-e02316

[90] Damato EG, Winnen CW. Cytomegalovirus infection: Perinatal

implications. Journal of Obstetric, Gynecologic, and Neonatal Nursing. 2002;**31**(1):86-92

[91] Chiopris G, Veronese P, Cusenza F, Procaccianti M, Perrone S, Daccò V, et al. Congenital cytomegalovirus infection: Update on diagnosis and treatment. Microorganisms. 2020;**8**(10): 1-17

[92] Leruez-Ville M, Ghout I, Bussières L, Stirnemann J, Magny JF, Couderc S, et al. In utero treatment of congenital cytomegalovirus infection with valacyclovir in a multicenter, open-label, phase II study. American Journal of Obstetrics and Gynecology. 2016;**215**(4): 462.e1-462.e10

[93] V'kovski P, Kratzel A, Steiner S, Stalder H, Thiel V. Coronavirus biology and replication: Implications for SARS-CoV-2. Nature Reviews. Microbiology. 2021;**19**(3):155-170

[94] Siddell S, Wege H, Ter Meulen V. The biology of coronaviruses. The Journal of General Virology. 1983;**64**(4): 761-776

[95] Jackson CB, Farzan M, Chen B, Choe H. Mechanisms of SARS-CoV-2 entry into cells. Nature Reviews. Molecular Cell Biology. 2022;**23**(1):3-20

[96] Meganck RM, Baric RS. Developing therapeutic approaches for twenty-first-century emerging infectious viral diseases. Nature Medicine. 2021;**27**(3): 401-410

[97] EMEA/H/C/005791 - Spikevax (previously COVID-19 Vaccine Moderna) EPAR Product Information: European Medicines Agency; [February 2022]. Available from: https://www.ema.europa.eu/en/medicines/human/EPAR/spikevax

[98] Harvey WT, Carabelli AM, Jackson B, Gupta RK, Thomson EC, Harrison EM, et al. SARS-CoV-2 variants, spike mutations and immune escape. Nature Reviews. Microbiology. 2021;**19**(7):409-424

[99] Tao K, Tzou PL, Nouhin J, Gupta RK, de Oliveira T, Kosakovsky Pond SL, et al. The biological and clinical significance of emerging SARS-CoV-2 variants. Nature Reviews. Genetics. 2021;**22**(12):757-773

[100] Knight M, Bunch K, Vousden N, Morris E, Simpson N, Gale C, et al. Characteristics and outcomes of pregnant women admitted to hospital with confirmed SARS-CoV-2 infection in UK: National population based cohort study. BMJ. 2020;**369**:1-7

[101] Dotters-Katz S, Hughes BL. Society for Maternal-Fetal Medicine (SMFM). COVID-19 and Pregnancy: What Maternal-Fetal Medicine Subspecialists Need to Know. Washington, DC: SMFM; 2020. Available from: https://www.smfm.org/covidclinical

[102] Karasek D, Baer RJ, McLemore MR, Bell AJ, Blebu BE, Casey JA, et al. The association of COVID-19 infection in pregnancy with preterm birth: A retrospective cohort study in California. The Lancet Regional Health – Americas. 2021;**2**:100027-100027

[103] Villar J, Ariff S, Gunier RB, Thiruvengadam R, Rauch S, Kholin A, et al. Maternal and neonatal morbidity and mortality among pregnant women with and without COVID-19 infection: The INTERCOVID multinational cohort study. JAMA Pediatrics. 2021;175(8): 817–826

[104] Cavicchiolo ME, Trevisanuto D, Priante E, Moschino L, Mosca F, Baraldi E. Italian neonatologists and

SARS-CoV-2: Lessons learned to face coming new waves. Pediatric Research. 2021;**91**(3):513-521

[105] Mitoulas LR, Schärer-Hernández NG, Liabat S. Breastfeeding, human Milk and COVID-19—What does the evidence Say? Frontiers in Pediatrics. 2020;**8**

[106] Vivanti AJ, Vauloup-Fellous C, Prevot S, Zupan V, Suffee C, Do Cao J, et al. Transplacental transmission of SARS-CoV-2 infection. Nature Communications. 2020;**11**(1):3572

[107] Centeno-Tablante E, Medina-Rivera M, Finkelstein JL, Rayco-Solon P, Garcia-Casal MN, Rogers L, et al. Transmission of SARS-CoV-2 through breast milk and breastfeeding: A living systematic review. Annals of the New York Academy of Sciences. 2021; **1484**(1):32-54

[108] Di Nardo M, van Leeuwen G, Loreti A, Barbieri MA, Guner Y, Locatelli F, et al. A literature review of 2019 novel coronavirus (SARS-CoV2) infection in neonates and children. Pediatric Research. 2021;**89**(5): 1101-1108

[109] Mantovani A, Rinaldi E, Zusi C, Beatrice G, Saccomani MD, Dalbeni A. Coronavirus disease 2019 (COVID-19) in children and/or adolescents: A meta-analysis. Pediatric Research. 2021;**89**(4): 733-737

[110] American College of Radiology. ACR Guidance on COVID-19 and MR Use. Available online: https://www.acr.org/Clinical-Resources/Radiology-Safety/MR-Safety/COVID-19-and-MR-Use; 2020

[111] Rosen H, Bart Y, Zlatkin R, Ben-Sira L, Ben Bashat D, Amit S, et al. Fetal and perinatal outcome following first and second trimester COVID-19 infection: Evidence from a prospective cohort study. Journal of Clinical Medicine. 2021; **10**(10):2152

[112] Stoecklein S, Koliogiannis V, Prester T, Kolben T, Jegen M, Hübener C, et al. Effects of SARS-CoV-2 on prenatal lung growth assessed by fetal MRI. Lancet Respiratory. 2022;**10**(4): e36-e37

[113] Gama MDP, Angelo Júnior JRL, Cunha-Correia C. Stroke in COVID-19 and pregnancy: A case report. Revista da Sociedade Brasileira de Medicina Tropical. 2021;**54**:e0301-e2021

[114] Sanders-Davis LJ, Ritchie J. Appendicitis with concurrent COVID-19 infection in a patient during the third trimester of pregnancy. BML Case Reports. 2021;**14**(6):e242651